D0406857

LOSE IT
FAST,
LOSE IT
FOREVER

LOSE IT
FAST,
LOSE IT
FOREVER

A 4-Step Permanent Weight Loss Plan from the
Most Successful "Biggest Loser" of All Time

PETE THOMAS

Foreword by
JILLIAN MICHAELS

AVERY
a member of Penguin Group (USA) Inc.
New York

Published by the Penguin Group
Penguin Group (USA) Inc., 375 Hudson Street, New York, New York 10014, USA •
Penguin Group (Canada), 90 Eglinton Avenue East, Suite 700, Toronto, Ontario M4P 2Y3,
Canada (a division of Pearson Penguin Canada Inc.) • Penguin Books Ltd, 80 Strand,
London WC2R 0RL, England • Penguin Ireland, 25 St Stephen's Green, Dublin 2,
Ireland (a division of Penguin Books Ltd) • Penguin Group (Australia), 250 Camberwell Road,
Camberwell, Victoria 3124, Australia (a division of Pearson Australia Group Pty Ltd) •
Penguin Books India Pvt Ltd, 11 Community Centre, Panchsheel Park, New Delhi–110 017,
India • Penguin Group (NZ), 67 Apollo Drive, Rosedale, North Shore 0632, New Zealand
(a division of Pearson New Zealand Ltd) • Penguin Books (South Africa) (Pty) Ltd,
24 Sturdee Avenue, Rosebank, Johannesburg 2196, South Africa

Penguin Books Ltd, Registered Offices: 80 Strand, London WC2R 0RL, England

Most Avery books are available at special quantity discounts for bulk purchase for sales promotions,
premiums, fund-raising, and educational needs. Special books or book excerpts also can be created
to fit specific needs. For details, write Penguin Group (USA) Inc. Special Markets,
375 Hudson Street, New York, NY 10014.

ISBN 978-1-58333-499-7

Printed in the United States of America
1   3   5   7   9   10   8   6   4   2

BOOK DESIGN BY TANYA MAIBORODA

While the author has made every effort to provide accurate telephone numbers, Internet addresses, and other contact
information at the time of publication, neither the publisher nor the author assumes any responsibility for errors,
or for changes that occur after publication. Further, the publisher does not have any control over
and does not assume any responsibility for author or third-party websites or their content.

PUBLISHER'S NOTE

CONTENTS

STEP THREE • YOUR PURSUIT

STEP FOUR • YOUR PURPOSE

FOREWORD

by Jillian Michaels

WHEN PETE THOMAS ARRIVED ON *THE BIGGEST LOSER* RANCH HE weighed over 400 pounds. He was one of the first contestants on *The Biggest Loser* to weigh that much. I remember telling Bob Harper that I wasn't sure what the results of training someone like Pete would be, but I was committed to giving my all to whip Pete and the other contestants into shape. The first time I met Pete I couldn't tell if he was actually "in it to win it." Not the cash prize, but his life. I knew Pete *needed* to win back his life, and I wasn't going to let him down. I believed in him until he learned to believe in himself. What I soon discovered was that Pete was equally committed—although I don't think he had any idea what he was in for.

Pete thought I was trying to kill him on the first day of filming for the show, but I knew he had to go somewhere he may have never gone before if he was going to change his health and his life forever. Two and a half hours into our workout on the first day, I challenged the contestants to a race, a hundred-yard dash. A wave of terror crossed over Pete's face, and remained there as I beat one contestant after another. When it was Pete's turn, I looked up at this six-foot-five giant and screamed at the top of my lungs, "Pete, if you don't beat me in this race, I'm going to pound you for another hour and a half!" Up until that moment, I'd never seen a guy that big run that fast. He was shaking and looked liked he was about to pass out, but he pushed through his fear and pain to beat me to the finish line. Never mind that I was running backward—Pete was fighting for his life and desperate to succeed. I don't know who was more surprised by his performance: Pete or me.

That was the beginning of many watershed moments for us on *The Biggest Loser*. As Pete lay there on the ground after winning—virtually unresponsive and barely able to talk—I remember giving him a hug and telling him, "Good job." That's when Pete said something to me I've never forgotten: "Just don't let me go back fat." At that moment I promised Pete that he wouldn't, and this book is the result of that promise.

When Pete was voted off *The Biggest Loser* Ranch, I told him that he needed to lose 100 pounds on his own, at home, if he expected to win the At-Home prize. He lost 102 pounds at home, bringing his total weight loss to an astonishing 185 pounds, and did indeed become the At-Home winner. Pete exceeded my wildest expectations, and his own, by keeping the weight off permanently. I can honestly say that Pete is no longer a fat person struggling to stay skinny. Pete truly believes that the new Pete—almost 200 pounds lighter than when I first met him—is the real Pete.

There's a kind of person on *The Biggest Loser* who just wants to be told what to do. Give me a packet of food to eat. Tell me how many push-ups to do in thirty seconds. That wasn't Pete. On the ranch, Pete would ask me questions and take notes. When he didn't understand something I said, he'd go away and research it on his own. His plan, this book, is the outcome of his search for those answers, and what he discovered along the way.

Pete has given a lot of thought on how to maintain your health once you've lost a significant amount of weight. He's taken many of the principles we talked about on the ranch and applied them to the pressure cooker of real life. I can truly say that Pete was one of my most dedicated students, and to prove it I keep inviting him to come and work with me on my projects. Why? Very simple. Pete kept the weight off long after the cameras stopped rolling. I like to show him off. He makes *me* look good.

I believe Pete's program is going to be a ladder for many people who need to move up to a new level in their lives. Let Pete's story inspire you to achieve your own goals and dreams. He's done it, and so can you. You are worth it, so put his actions into practice and see your life change in every imaginable way.

You really can Lose It Fast and Lose It Forever!

—Jillian Michaels, former *Biggest Loser* trainer and bestselling author of *Master Your Metabolism* and *Unlimited*

ACKNOWLEDGMENTS

I WOULD LIKE TO THANK MY CREATIVE TEAMMATE AND GHOSTWRITER, Randall Bonser, who took my words and stories and turned them into a very well-written book.

Rick Broadhead, our literary agent, who has guided us through turbulent waters, I can't thank you enough. Marisa Vigilante and all the folks at Avery Penguin, your vision, expertise, clarity, and hard work have all contributed to what this book has become.

I would also like to thank Team Thomas: Katrina, Wayne, Bob, Breanna, Kendall, Natashia, Amy, and the best business partner in the world, Anita Lane.

My LIF2 / SLIM U Families and all the folk I teach—you question me and challenge me to explain how I am successful at keeping the weight off. Because of you I am able to put on paper all the things I have learned and practiced over the years.

The Biggest Loser family—the casting directors, executive producers, my teammates and fellow cast members, contestants present and past, and most of all, Jillian, for seeding my mind with the possibilities of a new life.

Most of all, my Lord and Savior Jesus Christ, for strength and inspiration throughout my life. Where would I be without your unmerited favor?

INTRODUCTION
HOW MANY YEARS ARE YOU THROWING AWAY?

SIXTEEN. WHENEVER I GET DISCOURAGED IN MY WEIGHT LOSS JOURNEY, I think about that number. That's the number they gave me on *The Biggest Loser* Ranch. After Dr. Robert Huizenga, the show's physician, had done my medical assessment, he told me that if I stayed at my present weight—which was over 400 pounds—I would be cutting sixteen years off of my life.

What would you do with an extra sixteen years? Or even one extra year? Sixty percent of Americans are overweight. A staggering 30 percent of us are clinically obese. What events are we going to miss out on because obesity-related conditions cut our lives short?

Are you going to allow your bad health to rob you of amazing events that may happen in your life? Will your granddaughter be inaugurated the first female president but you won't live long enough to see it? Will your son play Carnegie Hall but heart disease will have put you in the ground before your time? Will my team, the Detroit Lions, finally win the Super Bowl but I'll miss it because I'll no longer be around? This book is an opportunity for you—an opportunity to take back your life and be there for those events that matter so much.

WHAT KIND OF DIETER ARE YOU?

I've been teaching people to lose weight with my program, Lose It Fast, Lose It Forever, for a number of years now. No matter where I teach it, I always start my classes with a "hook." Often it's a question or a series of questions to get my students' minds working, and to get the uncommitted to quit (more about this in Chapter 2).

Question number one: Why are you reading this book?

Here's another: How many diet books have you read?

Better yet: How many diets have you actually been on?

Chances are, this isn't your first rodeo. If you're like millions of other overweight people, you've ridden several different bucking broncos, and gotten thrown off all of them. Oh, I'm sure that if you're like me, you lost some weight on each plan. But—and believe me, I can relate to this—how much did you gain back? And how quickly did you gain it back?

I'm not making fun of you or trying to make you feel bad. Well, maybe a little. I poke fun at myself a lot, because I've tried so many diet plans, I could write a book on my failures over the years! But this is not a book about failure—this is a book about success. My success in keeping the weight off for more than seven years and counting after leaving *The Biggest Loser*. And your success, because you're finally going to lose that extra weight once and for all.

However, in my opinion, there are several types of dieters who should not read *Lose It Fast, Lose It Forever*. "What? He's telling me I shouldn't read his book? What's wrong with this guy?" Stay with me, I'll explain what I mean.

The Perpetual Dieter

This person reads diet book after diet book and collects all types of information. She reads blogs and articles and watches *The Biggest Loser* and buys every new exercise DVD. This person will buy gym memberships and equipment and may even ask everyone around her tons of questions about dieting and nutrition. She will work out at the gym for a couple weeks before quitting. The perpetual dieter is also the type who pops pills to lose weight. She tries and fails over and over again. For years. But she never actually works on the habits of success or follows a prescribed program through to its completion, so she never achieves any level of lasting success.

The You-Do-It-for-Me Dieter

These folks choose a variety of solutions—as long as they don't have to do the work themselves. For instance, they may choose bariatric surgery instead of behavioral change, without realizing that even after surgery there is a lot of hard work ahead to keep the weight off. As long as the hard work is done by someone else, sign them up. The fact is that you will not see health-related success without some effort on your part. The secret to weight loss success is developing daily habits that change the way you live. I tell my students, "It's impossible to make a lifestyle change if you don't really want to change your life." We will talk much more about this in Step 1. The bottom line is, if you want someone else to do the work for you, your weight loss will never be permanent.

The Pie-in-the-Sky Dieter

A few years ago, one of my students approached me after two weeks into my weight loss course—the ten-week course on which this book is based—and complained that she was dropping out of my class because the pace of her weight loss was *too slow*. "I've only lost four pounds," she whined. She missed the major fact that at that pace she could be expected to lose 100 pounds that year alone!

After asking her if she had written down her goals in the first class—which she hadn't—I could have told her to "stick with the program," and "hang in there for your health," and "we have not even covered exercise or delved deeply into nutrition yet." All those things would have been true. But more important, I sensed that she was simply an unrealistic dieter who wanted pie-in-the-sky results. She wanted a lot for a little. This person did eventually drop out of my class and I heard through social media that she had "tried Pete's class but it didn't work" for her. Imagine a young basketball player taking a clinic from Michael Jordan, then dropping out after two weeks because he couldn't dunk yet. I've seen many, many people gain their health back and see amazing results from Lose It Fast, Lose It Forever, but you have to be personally invested to see these results.

The Do-It-Tomorrow Dieter

This dieter has not really come to grips with the real reasons to lose weight. He is always starting next Monday or after the holidays. He has not experienced enough personal health issues or used enough insulin needles or taken enough medications or seen enough relatives die from heart disease to motivate him to start by going on a walk today.

As a matter of fact, this dieter probably would need to have the Angel of Death knocking at his door to make a real change. And even then he might ask, "Hey, can you come back tomorrow? The game is on." He may have been beaten down by life so much that he has lost his reason to live, so living healthy is an obscure thought.

ALL OF THESE people have one thing in common—they are dieters. Now let me tell you a secret.

At one point or another in my life, I fit all of these descriptions.

This book is not for any of these dieters. This book is for a different category of person: the one who is tired of all diets—period. You're tired of popping this pill or drinking that drink or eating this or that diet food and getting the temporary "fix" that comes with it. You've tried a lot of stuff, maybe even surgery in an attempt to bring your weight under control. But you've failed to some degree each time. And you're fed up with it all. Well, you've come to the right place, because I was tired also. I just wanted to stop dieting!

Diets are made to be followed. Life is made to be lived. I wanted to start living. Now I am living, and so can you.

FINDING THE "WHY"

I have spent the majority of my adult life as a severely obese man. I had to learn a lot of lessons to achieve my seven-plus years of excellent health. So you will excuse me when I say that my goal is not for you, the reader, to lose 10 or 15 pounds fast on my plan (although many of you will). Losing 10 or 15 pounds fast is no big deal. I've done that dozens of times, and you probably have as well. I am more concerned with you losing the weight forever. And to do that, you have to go deeper. You can't start this program without asking yourself, "Why?" Why are you overweight? And why do you want to lose weight forever? You have to start with a "why" and then set goals. I will help you with both of those, so don't worry. And of course you need to follow a really good plan tailored to your personal goals and life situation. Together we will develop that as well. It will take some work and commitment, but together we can do this. I'll tell you my "why" story if you tell yours.

THE ROOTS OF MY OBESITY

I lived in twelve cities before I was ten years old. My mother never seemed to be able to hold down a job or stay in one place very long. I got used to being on the move. And being hungry. One event stands out to me so clearly and painfully that when I close my eyes I feel like I'm back there. We were living in an apartment complex in the small town of Ypsilanti, Michigan. I must have been around five, because I was just learning how to tie my shoes.

It was summer, and I had recently received a Green Machine, a low-riding Big Wheel–type tricycle, and had finally figured out how to work the two little shifters. I was in little boy heaven. I could ride my Green Machine on the sidewalk around the parking lot, back and forth, in a little U shape for hours. That summer was going to be so cool!

I don't remember why, during what was shaping up to be the best summer ever, my mother told me she was leaving. She offered no explanation, only telling me that she had to go away for a little while. She was all I had—my whole world. I had never met my father, and to this day I have never even seen a photograph of him.

I didn't understand why my mother was leaving, but I did understand her instructions. She said I could continue to ride my Green Machine outside as much as I wanted. She left me no food but explained that three times a day I was to walk through the courtyard to the neighbors' house and ask them for something to eat. Then I was to return home and put myself to bed. Would you ever leave your five-year-old son by himself and tell him to beg food from a neighbor when he got hungry? I later found out that my mother struggled with a growing mental illness and could not see how her actions would affect me in so many ways.

Maybe this was the start of my struggle with food. It certainly was the beginning of my struggle for acceptance and belonging. When my mother came back after a week or so she brought a present: my little sister, Melay. I thought, "Wow, how cool! I have a little sister!" I was too young to realize my mom was pregnant, and we were estranged from our extended family, so I don't know if they knew about the new baby. But honestly, I was thrilled to have a little sister.

I would like to say this was the last time I was abandoned by my mother, but the story does not get any better. Less than two years later, the three of us had relocated to Detroit, to a nice big house on a quiet street. I was happy there, mainly because I could walk through our backyard straight onto a playground with a big cement turtle.

One day my mom told me she was going away again. I remember her teaching me how to heat up water in a pot and cook hot dogs for Melay and me. I remember thinking how long it took to heat up water on the stove, so I filled the sink with hot water from the tap and "cooked" the hot dogs in there instead.

To this day I do not know where my mom went, but this time she stayed away much longer. This time there was no neighbor to feed us. This time it was winter. And yes, this time the food ran out.

I remember waiting as long as I could, but finally I looked at my little sister and knew that we had to find food. I put on her hat and scarf and coat and boots, and mine as well. I walked out of the back door across the backyard onto the snowy playground toward the cement turtle. I distinctly remember seeing my mother's scarf on the turtle, even though I hadn't seen her for over a week. I reasoned that Mommy must be dead, because why else would she let the food run out?

As sad as that is, that may have been the best thing for me to think because I knew that we had to get moving. We had to find some food. And thankfully the first house we came to was not occupied by a child-molesting monster but rather caring people who took us in, fed us, and drove us to the police station that night. These events started my struggle with food. But the real struggle, as you can probably tell, went much deeper. It was a struggle for love. And unfortunately sometimes the two can be all mixed up together.

That was the day I began my journey in and out of the foster care system. Even though I was separated from my mother, her severe mental illness continued to impact my life. When I was eight years old, my mother actually found the foster home where I was staying and "kidnapped" me while I was at school and took me out of state. For some reason she did not take my sister, Melay, with us, and that was the last time I ever saw my sister. I don't know where she is, or even whether she's still alive.

As you can imagine, this kind of upbringing does not lend itself to learning good eating or any other habits. When we had food, I would wolf it down as fast as I could. And many times the food we had was not in the slightest bit healthy but was whatever greasy fast food we could afford. For a short period we lived in East Lansing, Michigan, where we attended a Catholic church, not because my mother was Catholic but because the church bulletins came with two-for-one Whopper coupons from Burger King. Sometimes she would tell me we were "fasting" when the truth was that we just had no money for food. To this day, when my stomach feels empty, I experience a vague sense of panic that manifests itself in the desire to fill myself up to overflowing. Fortunately I have learned this "why" for myself and I now know how to control it.

WHAT IS YOUR story? What causes you to overeat, or eat poorly, or engage in a behavior that's making you overweight? Because whether you know it or not, it is not just the taste of food that we love, it's what food represents. As a man who went homeless and hungry from time to time in my youth, I learned food represents safety. It represents normalcy. It represents all the things I didn't have when I was growing up.

To a person who has been divorced, food may stand for unconditional love. An extra serving of chocolate cake will never reject you. To a child who has been abused or seen abuse, food represents calm and quiet as you sneak away to your closet to enjoy your candy bars. Food helps us create an atmosphere of peace.

Food represents many things to many people, but it requires us to dig deep and discover what it means to us individually. After we discover what food means or represents in our lives, we have to take the next step and make sure we accurately understand the purpose of food. I'm going to ask you to explore these questions in Step 1: Your Power. But don't worry—you will not have to do this alone. There are very, very few things we humans do alone. Most things require teammates, partners, or an accountability structure of some type. I will help you build this team after reading Chapter 4. This journey will be difficult at times, but together we will make it through and see success.

I use the term "we" throughout this book for two reasons. The first is that, despite my seven years of weight loss success, I am still going through the process of forming lifelong healthy habits—I call them "Forever Habits." Forever Habits are repeated, positive behaviors that you've had in place for at least four weeks—behaviors that are readily adaptable in any and every situation. You'll know they're starting to become permanent when they've withstood at least one major challenge, such as eating well over the holidays or exercising when on vacation.

The second reason I use the term "we" is because long after you read this book, I will stay in touch with you and others in the Lose It Fast, Lose It Forever community through my social media. You will notice I use the acronym LIF2 to refer to Lose It Fast, Lose It Forever. I pronounce it "Life 2," because so many of my students have gained a new life through the tremendous weight loss they've achieved. You will hear some of their stories in the quotes at the beginning of each chapter.

THE FAST AND THE FOREVER

This is not a book of tips or tricks. I like to say, "Tricks are for kids. Education is for adults." We don't need tips. Nor do we need a temporary fix for the upcoming holiday party. You and I both need a life change. To truly change you must engage your most powerful weight loss weapon—your mind—to help you create Forever Habits that will guarantee your long-term success. This book will not give you all the answers. But this book will give you tools to find your own solution. This book will give you a plan that will work—whatever your situation, and no matter how much you want to lose. But you have to do the work. This is not a diet or a quick fix but a new way of living. You will Lose It Forever as you come to understand the mechanics of weight loss and develop healthy Forever Habits that you apply day in, day out, month after month. You will Lose It Fast as you apply those Forever Habits in a more aggressive manner.

Lose It Fast, Lose It Forever is broken up into four steps:

- Step 1: Your Power, in which you will learn to Master Your Mind. I will ask you to make a solid commitment to losing weight permanently, and then I will lead you through goal setting and team recruitment. We're going to make sure you employ the number one tool for successful weight loss: your mind!
- Step 2: Your Plan, in which you will learn to Manage Your Mouth and Multiply Your Muscles. This is the (lean) meat of the plan, if

you'll pardon my pun. We will study the mechanics of weight loss and use that knowledge to develop a Perfect Personalized Forever Meal Plan and a Perfect Personalized Forever Workout Plan. I have included sample menus and a workout plan to help you on your way. As you develop new eating and exercise habits to fit your lifestyle, you will start to see the pounds and the unhealthy behaviors melt away.

- Step 3: Your Pursuit, in which you will put it all together for a fast transformation. Do you have an occasion where you need to lose a number of pounds quickly? Or are you having a tough time with that last 15 or 20? I will help you "pursue" rapid weight loss with secrets and principles I learned while I was a contestant on *The Biggest Loser*— and after I returned home. I will help you make new goals and go after them aggressively using the same LIF2 principles you learned in the first two steps. I have included a sample menu and an intense 12-week workout plan to help you achieve these more time-oriented goals.

- Step 4: Your Purpose, in which you will enjoy your new life as you fulfill your true life's purpose in your new, healthier body. This is not just the "maintenance" step, it is the step where you celebrate your new life by passing your knowledge on to someone else. In this section we also talk about forgiveness and "getting back on the horse" if you have a bad stretch.

Some of you (primarily those of the perpetual dieter type) will be tempted to turn right to Step 3: Your Pursuit and try to implement the menu and exercise plans without reading Steps 1 and 2. Although you would see some "fast" weight loss, you probably wouldn't experience the "forever" part of the promise.

On the other hand, if you read through Steps 1 and 2, you'll have the knowledge to change your habits one at a time, which will build one success after another until you've actually lost a "Forever Five" or more, and in the process transformed your life. And once you change your life, weight loss is just around the corner. Once you've learned the basics of mental preparation, nutrition, and fat-burning exercise, then you'll be able to put it all together in Step 3 and watch those pounds come off more quickly than you ever thought they would. Like everyone who's come from *The Biggest Loser*, I advocate rapid weight loss for the sake of your heart and to bolster motivation. But I'm more concerned that you change your habits so you can live healthy forever.

And just a quick caveat here to calm down those of you who are nervous right now. "He wants me to move through this fast, but I'm too busy to attack it that quickly!" Relax. You can go through this program at whatever pace you want. Whether you need to lose 15 pounds or 150 pounds, the principles are the same. And whether you're a housewife from Florida or a *Biggest Loser* contestant in California, you both have to lose the pounds by creating one new Forever Habit at a time. So don't let the enormity of your goal get you uptight—just concentrate on the next habit and watch the next pound take care of itself.

YOUR SECRET WEAPON

In case you don't realize it, this plan is different from others because with this plan you have a secret weapon on your side: me. I've been there. Now I'm on the other side of *there*, throwing a life preserver back to you so that you can come over here to this side—the healthy side. The side of life where medications are reduced or dropped completely. Where clothes are bought in normal sizes at normal stores. Where you can sit in a regular airplane seat and not need a seat-belt extension. On this side, life is about pursuing your ultimate purpose and not just existing as a fat version of your real self. I'll be with you every step of the way, because I've been through just what you are experiencing. After all, forever is a long time.

So let us begin. Let's discover our why as well as the how so that together we can Lose It Fast, Lose It Forever.

STEP ONE
YOUR POWER

"There is so much misinformation out there. I realized that I only thought I understood what it took to lose weight, but I was doing everything wrong. LIF2 gave me the correct information, as well as the inspiration I needed. I lost 50 pounds, and continue to lose more! It is a lot easier to accept the information from someone who has been through the process, and a lot harder to make excuses."

—STEPHANIE, LIF2 STUDENT

CHAPTER

1

MASTER YOUR MIND

"PETE, IF YOU DON'T BEAT ME IN THIS RACE, I'M GOING TO POUND you for another hour and a half!"

Have you ever felt like dying was imminent? Maybe you've seen headlights coming straight toward you on an icy road or been on the top floor of a building during an earthquake. If so, you can relate to what I was feeling.

I was looking down at a tiny woman in a sleeveless T-shirt. Standing on her tiptoes she barely reached my armpits. At 401 pounds, I could have sat on her and squashed her like a bug. But I'd never been so afraid of somebody in my life. This wasn't just any woman screaming at me, this was Jillian Michaels, the famous and feared celebrity trainer. I was a few hours into my first day on NBC's *The Biggest Loser* and we had already been working out for two and a half hours.

To really understand why I thought I was close to death, let me set the scene: I am slowly running across a lush green polo field along with thirteen other obese people. I am filled with anticipation. I am ecstatic, thinking that I am about to embark on the adventure of a lifetime. From a distance, I run toward the voice of my new trainer, Jillian Michaels. This is day one on *The Biggest Loser* Ranch, and I can't imagine being anywhere else in the world. I am ready to be reborn. I am in fat heaven.

Then I actually meet Jillian.

And soon after that, I meet the pain.

I had thought that the very first day on *The Biggest Loser* Ranch would involve a little walking, a little stretching, maybe a trip over to the pond to watch the lilies float on the water.

Not exactly. That very first day, Jillian put us through two and a half hours of the most grueling, butt-kicking exercise you can imagine. We were doing a combination of push-ups, sit-ups, dumbbell presses, lunges, sprints with weights, squats, and more push-ups. It might have been halfway bearable if we had gotten some breaks in between. But we didn't get any breaks. No sitting down on machines, no resting, no bathroom breaks. The only break we got was when we staggered over to the side of the yard to throw up. Then we had to immediately get up and do it all over again.

I would like to point out that we contestants hadn't gotten fat by moving around a lot at home. We weren't "just a little out of shape." We had gone from completely sedentary to two and a half hours of intense exercise that very first day.

After two and a half hours of this sweaty, fat carnage, Jillian challenged us, "If you can beat me in a race, I'll cut the workout short and end it right here." She began to line up and race the other contestants over a flat stretch of land about a hundred yards long. She beat one after another.

Even while I was waiting my turn to race Jillian, my chest felt like it was on fire, I was light-headed, my vision was blurry, all my muscles were trembling, and I was close to fainting. I vividly remember thinking, "If I work out for even ten more minutes, I'm going to die." I realized that the outcome of this race would determine my next hour and a half, and possibly my entire life. I was committed to beating her. More important, I was committed to losing the weight necessary to become healthy again.

She said, "Go!" and we took off. I carried my 400-pound body down that stretch as fast as I could. I swung my sixty-inch belly back and forth, trying to build a little bit of momentum. It was not a pretty sight. Now, if you've been paying attention, you already know how the story ends from Jillian's foreword. But before I tell you the ending from my perspective, I want to explain where my commitment to succeed came from.

My rock-solid commitment had not magically appeared during that first killer workout. Nor had it come months before when I sent my first videotape in. It did not come when I drove to Indianapolis for my private interview with NBC's casting directors. It did not come when I flew out to California from Detroit to try out for the show. My strong commitment actually grew out of an emotional experience I had the very night before coming to the ranch.

AN END . . . AND A BEGINNING

We contestants had been secluded from each other in a hotel in Los Angeles for the previous ten days as we tried out for the show. Trying out involved some routine medical exams as well as a battery of psychological tests. I like to say that these psychological tests were to make sure the fat people wouldn't fly off the handle and try to strangle someone when we were deprived of our chocolate cupcakes. Finally those of us selected were told that we had made the show, and that we would be headed out to *The Biggest Loser* Ranch in vans that left at three in the morning. All night my mind had been flooded with restless thoughts and feelings of anticipation. We were told that there would be no phones allowed for the entire duration on the ranch, which could last as long as three months, so we were making our final calls to friends and family.

Around midnight, I received a phone call that would change my life. My aunt Lois, who lives in L.A., finally got ahold of me, after playing phone tag for a week. Having grown up in foster care, I had not had a lot of contact with my relatives, and I had not talked with this aunt for many years. I quickly told her the good news about being on the show, and then we started discussing the real reason that I had been trying to reach her.

For months prior to the show I had been trying to find information on my father, whom I had never known, and about whom my mother never talked. My aunt and I talked about my upbringing for more than two hours. Finally she told me that my father had died when I was just a little boy.

I was devastated. I had wanted my father, wherever he was, to share this life-changing experience with me when I found him. I had been imagining how proud he would be when we finally met up. Now I had to come to grips with the fact that I would have to do this without him. I now knew I needed to walk this road and conquer this enemy by myself. And for myself.

I knelt on the side of the bed in the room and began to speak to God. I said, "God, I don't know what is in store for me on this show. But I know that you blessed me to get here. So let's make a deal. I will do *whatever* they tell me to do, but Lord, just don't let me die." And with those words, I formed a rock-solid commitment to losing weight.

To really change your life, you have to really want to change it. No one can make you live differently. Well, they can, but the improvements won't be permanent unless you want it for yourself. I realized that night that I really wanted to change, and I was being given a precious opportunity to make a lasting difference if I could commit to taking advantage of the tools being offered. I have never regretted making that never-look-back commitment.

RACE TO THE FINISH

But that very first day on the ranch, my commitment was sorely tested. Here I was, barreling down to the finish line to try to cut the workout short after a grueling two and a half hours. I think I caused a small earth tremor in the surrounding mountains, but I ended up beating Jillian in that race.

I collapsed on the cement, barely conscious. Jillian was upset, as she had been planning on pounding us for a while longer. But finally she sat down on the ground and hugged me. As soon as I could speak, I told Jillian, "I prayed that I would get you as a trainer; just don't let me go back fat!" She reassured me by telling me, "You won't, babe, you won't."

Up until that point in my life, I had never been pushed so hard physically or emotionally. I felt like death was a real possibility at any moment, but giving up wasn't. I was willing to give my all to get healthy again. Even after I was voted off of the show, I was committed to gaining my life back. In fact, I was so committed that I continued to lose weight after I left the ranch, which allowed me to win the $100,000 At-Home prize in Season 2.

Now what about you? Yes, you. I am not going to ask you to go through anything half that hard over the next few months. But the question still remains: Are you really, really committed to becoming healthy?

MASTER YOUR MIND

You may wonder why I am not starting this program by talking about the food you need to eat, or the exercise you need to do to lose the weight. Those things are important, but there's something more important, and we have to take care of that before you can permanently change your eating and exercising habits. This step is called "Your Power" because your most powerful weight loss tool is your mind. Without plugging into that power source, you will never see permanent success. You could lose some weight, like all of us have, but without transforming your mind, permanent change will elude you.

Some people think you can Master Your Mind by flipping a mental switch and you'll immediately become a disciplined person capable of controlling yourself in every situation. But that's a myth—the mind doesn't work that way. If that were true, we'd all just go get an electric shock that made our brain behave every time we looked at a piece of fried chicken or chocolate cake.

Lasting change occurs when we come to the point where we understand that we need to change, and then apply a solution that makes sense to us. That involves a process of self-discovery, followed by searching out information, understanding why it's true, internalizing it, and applying it to our situation. If we do this a number of times, we will begin to form Forever Habits that point us toward healthy behavior, no matter where we find ourselves. It's like your ABCs—first we learn the letters, then we learn to put them together into words and sentences, then we use those sentences to communicate in any situation—even if we've never been in a particular location before. I like to say you take the information and turn it into application through systematic education, which allows you to make decisions in every new situation.

This kind of systematic education will help you make decisions in pressure situations. That's going to be important, because you won't need someone telling you what to do or how much to eat—you'll already know how and why to modify what is offered. And when you travel to a place without a gym or workout room, you'll know how to exercise in order to burn a specific number of calories. But you can only make those kinds of on-the-spot decisions if you Master Your Mind.

It kills me when I see overweight people blindly following crazy plans they see on TV or on the Internet and they have no idea why they work or even if they will be effective in their situation. They follow rules and special diets like sheep and then panic when they're in a situation that's "off the grid." They will drink shakes they've heard about on Facebook, without asking themselves, "Can I eat this way for the next month, let alone the next year?" Lose It Fast, Lose It Forever will help you Master Your Mind so that you can face food and life challenges with confidence and come through with flying colors. I know from teaching this for several years that some of you are still skeptical of the need to transform your mind. And it's true—if you only want short-term success, you can surround yourself with enough temporary motivation to achieve short-term goals. You can continue to ride the roller coaster, trying every new "miracle pill" and "fad diet" that hits the market. But if you want the kind of long-term success that this book promises, then you must Master Your Mind. And over the course of the next few chapters, we will learn to do just that.

KEY POINTS

- To get off the diet roller coaster, you've got to Master Your Mind first.
- It's time to ask the question: Am I really committed to becoming healthy this time?
- Forever Habits are formed as you take information and apply it through systematic education, which will give you confidence to make decisions in every situation.

CHAPTER 1 CHALLENGES

Tackling these challenges is going to take some time. Don't rush through them. You need to Master Your Mind, and these exercises are created to help you assess where you currently are and help stimulate your motivation.

Begin to Journal

We will start to explore our relationship with food. To do this we need to write down how certain foods make us feel and how the stress of the day affects our relationship with food. In the next chapter we will begin to keep an actual record of what we eat and drink, but for now we're just going to journal our thoughts and feelings. If it's helpful, you can download the LIF2 Success Journal that my students use from my website, www.PeteThomas.com (these questions and others are already in the journal when you download it). The discussion starters below will help you write meaningful entries in your journal for the first time. Write as much as you can so you can really explore your relationship with food.

- What are the main reasons you have gained extra weight (life events, lifestyle, upbringing, trauma, etc.)?
- Are you currently on a diet? If so, which one/type? What has been the result?
- If you are not currently on a diet, when was the date of your last weight loss program, and what was it?
- What is your biggest obstacle to losing weight?
- What kind of activities do you want to do when you lose the weight?
- How much weight do you want to lose?
- What is your current weight? What was it three years ago? What was it ten years ago? Have you ever been anorexic or bulimic? If so, please explain.
- List your exercise activity over the last thirty days (type of exercise, hours a week, estimate of intensity).
- What fears do you have about trying another weight loss program?
- Write down any final thoughts or insights.

Write Your Top 10 and Top 5 Lists

This is a fun motivational exercise to help you Master Your Mind. Start by writing down the "Top 10 Reasons I Want to Lose Weight" (these lists are also in the LIF2 Success Journal that you can download from www .PeteThomas.com, or feel free to use your own journal). These answers can be as altruistic as "I want to be around longer for my children" or completely superficial, like "I want to look sexy in that little black dress." You can put down more reasons than ten or you can list fewer reasons, but I prefer that you have right around ten, written in order of importance to you. You can give as much or as little explanation as necessary. It is going to be very important that you take the top three reasons, which I like to call your Personal Power Goals, and memorize them.

To drive the motivation even deeper into your gray matter, I want you to create two negative lists. One will be the "Top 5 Reasons I Hate Being Overweight." I don't usually encourage negative reinforcement, but it has been very effective in motivating certain students of mine. Follow that up with the "5 Things That Will Happen to Me if I Don't Lose the Extra Weight." These might be social consequences like "people won't want to sit next to me on an airplane" or medical consequences such as "I will develop diabetes."

Finish up with something positive as you write down the "Top 10 Things I Like About Myself." This doesn't have to have anything to do with your weight or body, although it certainly can if you feel that way. Getting in the habit of thinking positively about yourself will help you in the next chapter as you write your success statement. Complete these lists:

- Top 10 Reasons I Want to Lose Weight
- Top 5 Reasons I Hate Being Overweight
- 5 Things That Will Happen to Me if I Don't Lose the Extra Weight
- Top 10 Things I Like About Myself

"If you do Pete's plan you will lose weight, and it can change you from the inside out. I think as women we seem to put everyone in our life first. I never put myself on the to-do list, but I have learned to make myself a priority. I have lost 60 pounds doing this program and I am hoping to lose another 40 more. I have gone down from a size 24 to a 16. I have lost over 40 inches of fat. This program has saved my life."

—KENDALL, LIF2 STUDENT

CHAPTER

COMMIT OR QUIT

"YOU DID WHAT?"

My friend was looking at me incredulously. "You put your dining room table and chairs out on the roadside?"

I nodded my head. "And I put a sign that said 'Free' on it," I continued.

"Why would you do that?"

"Because I want to prove that I am committed to losing weight." I thought at the time that this made perfect sense. I had just spent $5,000 on two pieces of exercise equipment that I put in my dining room right where the dining room table and chairs formerly were.

I'll tell you how the story ends in a little bit. But first I want to make something very clear.

THIS BOOK COULD BE DANGEROUS TO YOUR HEALTH

I want you to think about your commitment level right now, before you read any further in this book. Are you committed to losing weight forever by changing one habit at a time, over and over, until you achieve your weight loss goals? Here is my challenge:

You need to either commit . . . or quit.

This may surprise you, but it's actually dangerous for you to be reading this and not be committed. Here's why. Have you ever lost five pounds, only to gain six back? I have. That's because as we begin to lose weight, our bodies send out signals by way of hormones that prime us to gain back all the weight we've lost, plus some extra.

The design of our bodies is amazing. When you begin to lose weight, your body thinks it might be going into starvation mode and it becomes anxious to gain all the weight back—and more—to protect itself. All your body knows is that it's not getting the same amount of fuel it used to get, and for a while it is going to resist you. Imagine your body talking after you lose some weight: "This is only temporary. As soon as we drop this new healthy lifestyle, I am going to try to pack on even more fat than we had before." This is what other programs don't tell us. They just let us ride the bathroom-scale roller coaster until we're thoroughly frustrated.

Don't be frustrated—you can do this. We're not focusing on the *what* anymore—that giant mountain of 25 or 30 or 100 pounds. We're focusing on the *how*—that next small step or Forever Habit that will lead to the next pound we need to shed. And I promise, your body will adapt. This will stop feeling like a "diet"—because it isn't—and start feeling like a healthy life, which it is.

MY PROMISE TO YOU

Here is my promise to you: At the end of reading this book, if you've made a commitment to following my principles, you will know nearly everything necessary to lose as much weight as you want, one Forever Habit at a time. You will never again have to ask the question "How do I lose weight?" I can assure you that you will have all the building blocks necessary to lose weight and live a much healthier life than the one you are currently living.

The real question is "Will I be committed to losing the weight?" While I will give you all the tools necessary, I cannot make you do the work necessary to lose the weight. Now I know what some of you are saying, "But, Pete, I am committed. I bought this book, didn't I? I put my money where my mouth is, and I am ready to go forward."

Please—don't even talk to me about spending money and saying you are committed.

COMMITMENT OR CLOTHES HANGERS?

Remember that expensive exercise equipment I mentioned in the opening of this chapter? I bought that in 2004, the year before I was cast on *The Biggest Loser*. I placed those two beautiful pieces of chrome and vinyl in my dining room, where they would be the center of attention.

I seriously thought I was committed to exercise. I walked on that treadmill every day for 30 days. After losing 10 pounds, I was frustrated, disgusted, and mad. I realized that I could have lost 10 pounds if I had just skipped dinner on Friday nights for a couple of weeks. I was so disappointed that I ditched that exercise program and went on to gain back those 10 pounds and then 10 more. Those two pieces of equipment became nothing more than expensive clothes hangers, the ironic backdrop for my *Biggest Loser* audition video later that same year.

Now, it's true that some equipment is going to be necessary for success in my program. Don't worry; the stuff is not expensive. At the end of this chapter in the Challenges section, I have included an equipment list, which includes measuring spoons, a digital scale to weigh food portions, a heart rate monitor, and a few other items.

The sad truth is that just because you spend some money on something does not mean that you are committed. And just because you start something does not mean that you are going to finish. The true test of your dedication will be the commitment of something much more valuable than money.

MORE VALUABLE THAN MONEY

The one factor I cannot control in your life is time. Time is our most precious asset and the one that is hardest to part with. I encourage you right now to take stock of your life and determine within yourself that you are important enough to spend whatever time is necessary to get to a healthier weight, forever. Do not make this decision lightly, because there are no shortcuts to lasting weight loss. Pills and miracle berries cannot keep us thin. Even people who undergo bariatric surgery don't get a free ride— they have to change their lives once they come out from under the knife. Don't worry, I'm not going to make you spend a lot of money on special foods or expensive exercise equipment, but we do have to spend our most precious asset, our time, if we want to shed those pounds forever.

This isn't going to be easy. Your employer needs you, your spouse or significant other needs you, your kids need you, your worship community and social groups need you, and yes, even your siblings and parents need you. I say this because you will have a tendency to say, "I've got too many responsibilities to spend all this time on weight loss."

I know the feeling. There was a time when I thought I was the center of the world, too.

I used to think, like many of you, that everything around me would fall apart if I was not there. I was sure that no one could manage without me. My church, my home, my family. They all needed me. So I let the most important thing in my life go. I let *me* go. And my weight soared to over 416 pounds with 50 percent body fat and a sixty-inch waist.

But then I went away for two and a half months to *The Biggest Loser* and I found something out. Nobody really needed me! I mean, I was important to all of my circles of influence, but they could all manage without me.

At the time, I operated my church's sound system a couple of times a week. Lo and behold, to my surprise, when I went away to *The Biggest Loser*, my church kept going on and having services without me. The nerve of some people! My role at the church was filled by the next warm body.

My friends told me before I left how much they would miss me while I was away at the ranch. Well, wouldn't you know it, not one of them took the time to write and mail a letter to me. Actually, that's not true.

One of them did write me a letter, but he is a writer by occupation so I am not sure I should even count him.

Of all the things I thought revolved around me, nothing really did! I know many of you feel like your world revolves around you, but I am willing to bet that everyone in it could get along fine without you if you take some time to invest in yourself.

You may be the caregiver in your family. In fact, one reason you may be overweight is that you take care of everyone else's needs before your own. That's what Shay Sorrells, a *Biggest Loser* contestant from Season 8, realized. After Shay stepped on the scale during week one, she said, "It made me realize that after twenty-nine years living to fix my mom, I spent twenty-nine years breaking myself." Maybe you can relate to that statement. Guess what? Your family and friends will learn to manage without you while you spend time becoming healthy. The question is, Can you let your family grow and learn to manage without you while you still have a choice in the matter? Can your family give you some time off for working out, or preparing meals for a whole week, or keeping a daily diary, or simply taking a couple of minutes each and every evening to de-stress? It's like the flight attendants on an airplane say in the safety instructions before you take off—secure your own mask before you help others with theirs. You really can't take care of anyone else if you don't take care of yourself first.

The bottom line is, you must focus on you for once in your life! Your alternative is not pretty—you can neglect yourself and continue dragging around that extra weight until you become a burden to those around you. Or if you are like I was and are among the 30 percent of Americans who are truly obese, you can simply die early from an illness related to your poor health. I promise you everyone will manage without you once you're in your grave.

But maybe death is so abstract it does not scare you, so let's make it a little more simplistic. Keep going the way you're presently going, taking care of everyone else around you, pick up 40 to 80 pounds over the next couple of decades, and watch your spouse divorce you for someone skinnier or your employer dump you to lower health insurance premiums. Then the fact that you spent time on everyone but you will reveal the shortsightedness of your actions.

The truth is, you will spend time on your health regardless of your diet and exercise habits. The choice of when you spend the time is up to you. One option is to voluntarily spend time preventing health issues from occurring by taking the time to practice good nutrition and exercise. Or you will be forced to spend the same amount of time running back and forth to doctors' appointments, picking up prescriptions from the pharmacist, going to dialysis, or ordering diabetic supplies.

When will you take the time? The choice is yours. Spending time on yourself is one of the most selfless things you can do. A better you means everyone around you is better off.

So here is the first commitment that we need to make: Commit to setting aside a portion of your day each and every day over the next several weeks for you. Time is like money; if you don't plan to put some aside, chances are you won't have any left for yourself. Students ask me, "How much time should I set aside for myself?" I tell them, "It's going to be different for everybody." For instance, I work out for an hour a day, and I also write in my journal for about fifteen minutes a day. That is sacred "me time." Some people may only have an hour to carve out, so you're going to have to figure out how to use that hour based on your goals. A chef who wants to lose weight doesn't have to spend time learning how to cook; he already knows how to flavor food with herbs and spices. On the other hand, someone who doesn't know how to cook is going to have to spend some "me time" learning to cook differently.

The bottom line is that you're going to have to spend as much time as you need to get healthy. Do you already exercise? Good, you may only need to add on a little bit more time. Do you spend every minute of your day caring for someone else? You may need to carve out time to retrain yourself to get rid of bad habits. For some people, writing may be a burden, but talking to a coach or mentor would be very helpful. Every person has different needs and goals, so "me time" is going to vary. It's more important to start carving out a chunk of time right away rather than worrying about how much is the right amount. You will understand your needs more thoroughly as you work through the program. Throughout the course of this book, you are going to have to digest a lot of information. More important, you are going to have to implement a lot of information. Don't get anxious—I know that we can do this. If I did it, you can, too. My motto is also my motivator: There's a Winner Wi*thin* You!

AN APPOINTMENT WITH YOURSELF

It's vitally important that you clear some time every day to work on you. You need to put some "me time" right into your schedule. Yes, write it down or type it into your calendar. From 4:00 to 5:00 in the afternoon, or 6:00 to 7:00 in the morning, or whenever works best for you. At first, you're going to spend time journaling, studying, reading, praying, doing whatever it takes to get your mind in the right place to change *you*. Eventually this will turn into exercise and food preparation time, but for now I just want you to make a date with yourself each and every day. As the business gurus say, if you fail to plan, you are planning to fail.

JOURNAL YOUR JOURNEY

In the Challenges section at the end of Chapter 1, I asked you to download the LIF2 Success Journal from my website, www.PeteThomas.com. If you don't have access to a computer, create your own LIF2 Success Journal. I introduced you to the concept of journaling about food by asking some pointed questions. I hope you found this rewarding and helpful. I want you to start writing about your relationship with food on a regular basis so that you can be aware if you've got a food fixation or if you eat when you're stressed, or if something else is going on. You can bring a lot to the surface just by recording your reactions to what you've eaten.

I also want you to record what you are eating, and when, in your journal. Make this "food journal" a regular part of your journaling. A food journal is simply a record of everything that goes into your mouth. Yes, everything! That includes both solid food and liquids. You will be surprised at how many calories a day you consume in the form of sodas, shakes, alcoholic drinks, white chocolate lattes, condiments, and so on.

For me to develop new Forever Habits so that I could Lose It Forever, I had to become aware of the food I was eating. You're not going to make any changes yet; you're just keeping a record. Most of my students come back to class after starting this journal just shocked and amazed at all that they eat, with snacks and extra meals thrown in. You may be shocked as well. But it will be a good education.

Getting a handle on what we're eating is going to lead to the next steps described in Step 2: Your Plan, so we need to get started now. We're getting closer and closer to that goal of creating new Forever Habits.

MOVE SOMETHING

We will talk more extensively about exercise in Step 2: Your Plan. In Chapter 13 you will even find a number of workouts for people with different experience levels and goals. But right now, today, I need you to take time for yourself and start getting in some light exercise just as a way to get moving. I will explain what I mean, but first things first. Before you take part in any nutrition or exercise program, you need to talk to a medical professional about any limitations that you might have. Ask your doctor for permission to participate in strenuous daily physical exercise in the form of low-impact, high-intensity activities based upon your heart rate. In this step of the program, I'm not going to ask you to start sweating too hard. You're coming into a commitment to weight loss by dipping your toe in and checking out the water. But I do want you to take time for yourself by starting to move around if you haven't been moving around too much on your own. I'm not talking about walking from your car to the door of the mall; I'm talking about light exercise.

If you haven't begun to exercise, then taking "time for me" may mean you need to start walking for thirty minutes a day. This will introduce you to the concept of cardiovascular exercise, but it's not too strenuous. As you progress, you may want to follow my Get Off the Couch or Die— Absolute Beginner 6-Week Workout Plan that you will read about in Chapter 13.

If you already exercise, I want you to increase the intensity a little bit. If you're going to the gym and working out, step it up just a little bit to begin with and try to build up your "me time" in the gym by five minutes a week. Don't worry, I'll teach you how to really use exercise to Lose It

Fast in Step 3, but for now, I just want you to start working that heart a little bit in the form of walking thirty minutes a day or by increasing your exercise a bit at a time.

DE-STRESS

We talked a little bit in the Introduction about how our relationship to food causes some of us to have food issues. Many people relieve stress by eating. And often our "comfort foods" are the very foods that are sabotaging our health. So whatever measures we can take to relieve stress—the right way—will help us.

We need to find a time every night to just relax and de-stress. This will be "me time" in which we can unwind from the day's demands and let the workload, the pressures of raising kids, and the expectations of others just melt off. Reading a book during this time helps many people. I often journal during my de-stressing time to help myself unwind. However we do it, let's make sure we take "time for me." That's going to make us a better me for everyone else.

THIS IS NOT A DIET

One of the main things I have learned from teaching other students these very principles is that you cannot view this program as a diet but rather a life change. This is about forever. There are no fad diets here. No fad workouts. No miracle surgeries. No magic berries.

Lose It Fast, Lose It Forever offers something that will actually help you lose pound after pound for life—a tremendous amount of helpful information based on my experience on the ranch, as well as the research that I have done into the science of weight loss since I came back home.

Initially my research and reading was all for selfish reasons. I was simply desperate to keep the weight off. I wanted to learn why the principles taught on the ranch were successful. I also wanted to know why many dieters—and contestants—couldn't manage to keep the weight off once they had lost some. I lost 185 pounds during my time on the show, and I've kept the weight off for over seven years.

But it doesn't matter how much you know if you don't commit to taking action. You've got to make a decision to commit or quit today. If you are ready to change your life and regain your health, one pound at a time, then you will need to take a few action steps.

KEY POINTS

- Pete's challenge: Either commit . . . or quit.
- The true test of commitment is not money dished out but time spent on getting healthy.
- Lose It Fast, Lose It Forever is not a diet but a series of Forever Habits strung together to form a healthy life.
- By keeping a regular food journal in your LIF2 Success Journal, you are taking the first step in changing the way you eat forever.

CHAPTER 2 CHALLENGES

Commit to This Program

It's time to put your commitment down in writing. Answer the following questions in your LIF2 Success Journal to help you define your commitment to success in this weight loss venture.

1. Why did you buy this book? Please explain.
2. Let's assess some weight loss programs based on your experiences:
   - Make a chart with three columns and list the weight loss/diet programs you have tried in the left column (formal and/or informal programs). You can download this chart from www.PeteThomas .com if you like.
   - Take this chart and rate your past programs on a scale of 1 to 5 in the middle column, 1 being the least successful and 5 being the most successful.
   - In the third column, write why each program did or did not work for you.
3. What does commitment mean to you? What have you successfully committed to in the past?
4. Are you seriously committed to this program?

Write Your "Me Time" into Your Calendar

Don't just set aside time in your head. Put it into your calendar as if it were an appointment with your boss. Don't let other commitments squeeze out the time you spend pursuing your health.

Begin Keeping a Food Journal

You've already begun to write your thoughts and feelings about food in your journal. Now write down everything that goes into your mouth in your journal. This includes both solid foods and drinks of any kind. Keeping a food journal leads into one of the main points in Step 2: Your Plan, so do not skip this.

Get Medical Permission if You Don't Already Have It

Most people will be cleared to begin exercising immediately by their physician, but people with heart conditions will want to get any advice or restrictions their doctor has for them before they begin.

Start Walking Thirty Minutes a Day

If you don't presently exercise—and I'm not talking about playing ball in the backyard with the kids—start to walk for thirty minutes, either on the treadmill or around the block. This will introduce you to the rigors—and pleasures—of exercise slowly. If you already exercise, work out harder and start to increase your workout time by five minutes a week.

De-Stress

Take time every night to relax and de-stress. Maybe you can do this through your journaling. Maybe you'll read a book. Maybe the daily walk will do the trick. But begin to take some "me time" to relax.

Buy the Proper Equipment

If you are truly committed to losing those pounds forever, purchasing these items will be necessary to your success:

- Measuring supplies: You will need a digital scale that measures small amounts and a set of measuring spoons and measuring cups.

- A heart rate monitor with chest strap. This measures your heart rate and tracks your calories burned. Avoid versions without chest straps, because in my experience they're not as accurate.

- A good pair of running shoes, preferably purchased from a running store. The experts at a running store will watch how you walk and pick shoes according to your size and gait. I would never buy something as important as shoes from a store that also sells diapers or food.

- An easy-to-use, thorough calorie counter. This can be a book, a website, or an app on your smart phone. This invaluable tool will help you figure out the number of calories contained in various food portions, as well as the number of calories in common restaurant foods.

- A gym membership. Although this is not mandatory, many people find it easier to get away from home and work out in an atmosphere of like-minded individuals. Memberships can often be purchased for as low as $10 a month if you do some research. Prices may vary depending on where you live.

- Several good home workout DVDs. These will add variety to your workout and ensure that you get a workout when the weather is too nasty to go out. These DVDs need to be very intense—the harder the better. It's easy to make a challenging workout easier by doing your own modifications (more about this in Chapter 12), but it's difficult to make an easy DVD workout more intense. There are many good workout DVDs on the market, but don't just go get the latest fad program—make sure it provides an intense workout.

- Home exercise equipment, such as dumbbells and resistance bands. You will need something in the light, medium, and heavy range. I don't mean 2, 4, and 8 pounds—those are all in the light range. I usually recommend women start with 10-, 15-, and 25-pound weights, and men start with 15-, 20-, and 30-pound weights.

"I honestly always wanted to lose weight, but had tried so many things and failed that I didn't find it realistic. When I first started LIF2 I was 235 pounds. Today I am currently at 182.4 pounds, so I have lost 52.6 pounds. This program has definitely changed my attitude, because for once I believe that I can actually achieve the goals that I am setting for myself. It has changed my self-confidence: I feel beautiful and I am worth it!"

—JACQUATA, LIF2 STUDENT

CHAPTER

3

SET THE RIGHT GOAL

"WHOSE TWO-SISTER SUIT IS THAT?"

I was standing in front of a glass display case during the first week of filming on *The Biggest Loser*. Inside the display case was an outfit for every one of the contestants. Of course, none of us could fit the clothes yet. They were the outfits we wanted to wear when the show was over.

I had asked for a replica of the very classy white wool suit worn by one of the actors in the movie *Soul Food,* but the white suit I saw in the display case was nothing like it. Oh, by the way, have you met the two sisters I was referring to—Poly and Ester? We used to wear a lot of two-sister, or polyester, clothes back in the 1970s. My polyester "goal suit" at the ranch certainly was not wool—it was more *Miami Vice* than *Soul Food*. But in this case it was, literally, the thought that counted.

We were learning to set goals. Not vague goals like we had always set before, like "I want to lose a few inches" or "I want to be more attractive." No, we were being forced to get specific with our goals—hence the outfit we wanted to wear when we left the show.

I believe that there are two critical things that we have to get in place before we can begin to lose weight successfully. One is having great teammates, which we'll talk about in the next chapter. The other is setting great goals.

A great goal will keep you focused. A great goal will keep you encouraged. A great goal will also keep you motivated. It's easy to start a diet strong, not so easy to finish it strong. That's where a great goal will help us. I originally set a goal to lose 140 pounds because that would have put me at 265, which is what I weighed in my second year of college. You can set a goal using a healthy weight chart at your doctor's office, or you can go to www.PeteThomas.com to find a chart with a healthy weight for your body type.

I tell my students, "Having a goal of losing weight is stupid." When they look at me with shocked expressions, I explain, "You've set that goal before. Lots of times. I want your goal to be achieving a healthy weight and maintaining that for the rest of your life." It's like following a new equation with your life: Different Goals = Different Focus = Different Habits.

How much weight do you want to lose, and by what date? I promise, we'll get back to the one Forever Habit at a time very soon. But we need to establish a "finish line" so we can celebrate when we reach our long-term goal.

So how do we set a great Lose It Forever goal in weight loss? Simple. Your goal needs to be S.M.A.R.T.

MAKE A S.M.A.R.T. GOAL

S.M.A.R.T. is an acronym used in business settings to help people make better goals. I've adapted the acronym to help my students create weight loss goals. Your forever weight loss goal needs to be Specific, Measurable, Aggressive, Realistic, and Time-Based.

Specific

The "S" in S.M.A.R.T. stands for Specific. How much weight do you ultimately want to lose? I wanted to lose 140 pounds when I was cast on *The Biggest Loser*. At the time, I weighed in at a svelte 401 pounds. By the time I was voted off, I had shed 83 pounds of that, so my "at home" goal was to lose around 60 pounds before the live show finale. Like I have said before, I did this by creating Forever Habits that would help me Lose It Forever while applying those habits very aggressively to help me Lose It Fast. But as I began my journey, I knew specifically how much weight I wanted to lose in the long run.

Your goal needs to be specific, too. Ask yourself, "How much weight do I want to lose overall?" In the Challenges section, I'm going to ask you to write that specific number down.

Measurable

Next, our goals need to be Measurable. The process of measuring our weight loss and habits adopted will help keep us motivated. We want to journal our journey each and every step of the way so that we can track our progress toward success. And to track our progress, it has to be measurable.

What do I mean by that term? Measurable is the opposite of vague. Let me give it to you this way: A measurable goal is quantitative, not qualitative. A qualitative, or vague, goal is "I want to be thinner" or "I want to be more attractive to my spouse." There is nothing wrong with those goals, except that you won't know when you get there! Those goals are not all measurable. "I want to lose 25 pounds" is measurable because you're aiming for a number you can see on a scale. "I want to go down two dress sizes" is measurable.

The reason it has to be measurable is because we are going to actually measure our progress. You need to weigh yourself weekly and record your progress. You'll begin by taking your initial measurements in the Challenges section at the end of this chapter, and then continue to weigh yourself weekly to mark your progress. Each time you lose a couple of pounds or adopt a new Forever Habit, I want you to come and tell us how you did it at PeteThomas.com. It's a little early to talk about short-term goals that turn into Forever Habits, because we haven't covered nutrition and exercise yet, but I'll give you a few examples. A short-term goal after reading Chapter 6 might be, "I am going to start drinking diet soda or water" or "I am going to have a salad with every meal." A short-term goal you might set after reading Chapter 11 might be, "I'm going to exercise for thirty minutes, six days a week." Those are very specific, measurable short-term goals that will lead to Forever Habits.

Aggressive

Your long-term goal should also be as Aggressive as your schedule allows. There is no reason to drag out this weight loss for three or four years. Shedding the weight quickly will be good for your heart and your motivation.

The Biggest Loser has proven that quick weight loss is possible. However, if we are going to have an aggressive goal, the key will be dedicating "me time" every day to eating properly, exercising, and journaling in order to get the weight off in a steady, healthy way while implementing new Forever Habits to keep it off forever.

After I was voted off the show, I had to revise my goals to make them slightly less aggressive. After all, I wouldn't have the trainers around me all the time, and more important, I wouldn't have the same kind of free time. But I resisted the temptation to totally *weaken* my goal. I determined that if I could find the two and a half hours a day in my schedule, then I could still achieve my aggressive weight loss goal. That's how I lost 102 of my 185 pounds on my own in approximately six months.

Your goal is probably not that aggressive, but I want you to approach it with that much confidence. How aggressive should your goal be? That depends on how much you want to lose, and how quickly. In Chapter 10 we will discuss the F.I.T.T. (Frequency, Intensity, Time, Type) principle, which will give you an idea of how much you can lose in a certain amount of time, given your intensity level. Guidelines for healthy weight loss will always be dependent on how closely you adhere to the principles of the program. If you adhere strictly to the principles of LIF2, you can expect to lose between 1 and 2 percent of your body weight a week. This is still on the aggressive side—that is the kind of weight loss I see at my boot camps, and the kind of weight loss you will see if you follow the guidelines in Step 3: Your Pursuit. If you don't need to lose 1 to 2 percent of your body weight a week, you would not set that kind of aggressive goal and perhaps more modestly would plan to lose 1 to 2 pounds each week.

Realistic

Your goal also needs to be Realistic. The concept of realistic has been redefined by *The Biggest Loser*. Each week the world can now see that through proper eating and intense, vigorous exercise, we can lose an incredible amount of weight in a relatively short time. I realize that this "reality" show is not completely realistic, as the contestants are removed from their daily routine, but the principles do work in real life. I know this because I lost a majority of my weight at home after I left the ranch.

What we really have to think about is how much actual time we can dedicate to reaching our weight loss goals. If we can only exercise a half hour a day, it's going to take a little longer to reach our long-term goals, unless we put in a lot of work on the nutrition side. That's fine, but let's just be realistic about reaching that goal. Shedding 1 percent of your body weight a week is very possible, but it depends on how much time you're actually going to put into it. As I mentioned before, when we talk about the F.I.T.T. principle in Chapter 10, you'll have a clearer idea of how much you can expect to lose based on a number of variables that differ from person to person.

Time-Based

Finally, the "T" in S.M.A.R.T. means that our weight loss goals need to be Time-Based. By what date do you want to accomplish your goal? Is there a special occasion for which you want to lose the weight, like swimsuit season or a wedding? That will determine how aggressively we pursue our first pound, and then the second, and so on.

One of my students wanted to lose weight for her daughter's summer wedding. She wanted to look good in that special dress and in those keepsake photos. By first learning and then diligently working toward her goal, she lost 44 pounds and looked fantastic in her dress and learned the principles necessary to keep it off forever. You, too, will create a concrete, time-based long-term goal based on your particular circumstances and motivations.

CREATE A PERSONAL SUCCESS STATEMENT

A part of the process that I went through to master my mind involved changing the way I thought about myself. Changing my mind-set involved saying new and better things to myself. So often we allow the negative words of others to become our daily reality. Past words and current situations are not an indicator of future possibilities, unless we believe them to be so. As I began to set goals, I began to change the way I thought about myself by changing what I said to myself about myself and my goals. Let me repeat that:

I began to change the way I thought about myself by changing what I said to myself about myself and my goals.

I strongly believe that creating an emotional connection with your goals will help you achieve them. One way I have done this is by creating a Personal Success Statement. I have several of them, and I keep myself on track by getting up every morning and repeating one. Some examples: "Winners Do Daily What Others Do Occasionally" and "There's a Winner Wi*thin* Me." (Get it? Wi*thin*?) My primary success statement is, "I feel sexy, strong, and great as I maintain my weight at or around 238." That statement really helps keep me focused. Because it rhymes, it's easy to remember and helps me focus on the message.

I want you to use a Personal Success Statement to stay focused, too. You've heard my success statement. What's yours? For example, you could say, "I'm feeling more alive and satisfied as I weigh in at or below 155." You can begin to say this even if you currently weigh in at 255.

Your statement will be even more powerful if it is written as what I call a personalized, positive, present tense affirmation. I discovered that my old weight loss goal, "I want to lose 140 pounds," seemed impossible and it negatively affected my focus. I went through several adjustments and eventually settled on "I feel sexy, strong, and great as I maintain my weight at or around 238." Notice I don't say "I *hope* to feel great" or "I *want* to maintain my weight." It's both *positive* and *present* tense and mentions my goal (238 pounds) as well as describes how I will feel (great) when I reach my personal goal (maintaining my weight). I always try to put a positive emotional spin on my goals to help convince my mind that I can do whatever I set out to do.

Together we will walk through creating a Personal Success Statement in the Challenges section.

THE "BEFORE" IN BEFORE AND AFTER

People have often asked me, "Pete, how in the world could you stand up there practically naked in front of the entire world and have that big old belly just hanging out?" The reason I could allow myself to take that "before" picture was because I knew that a great "after" picture was coming. I was so confident that I would lose weight that before *The Biggest Loser* ever aired I took "before" pictures of myself. It was 2003 and I knew that I would one day lose so much weight that no one would recognize me. I just had no idea how it would happen. Then I ended up on *The Biggest Loser* and lost the weight in front of a few million people. Now even more people can see my amazing transformation on the cover of my book.

Do you have confidence that you will lose weight and keep it off permanently? Real confidence? Well, guess what—it's your turn to show the world that you can do this. (You knew this was coming, didn't you?) To really add some "weight" to your goal setting, I want you to take some "before" pictures. Preferably several of them. I will explain this in more detail in the Challenges section.

CREATE A REWARD SYSTEM

At the beginning of this section I explained my very concrete reward for losing weight. I visualized myself wearing a beautiful white suit—much nicer than the fake suit they used on the show—and I made sure my very first day home from the ranch, I bought it and wore it around to see my loved ones. That was my reward for all the hard work and sacrifice.

Now it's your turn. What will you do for yourself once you reach your goal? Do you have a dress or a bathing suit you want to fit back into? I want you to purchase your goal outfit, if you don't already own it. If you can't purchase it, find a picture of it on the Internet and print it out. Next, place the goal outfit or a picture of it somewhere prominently in your home as a mental reminder of what you're shooting for. Tape your Forever Goals next to it to remind yourself of how you're going to achieve that goal outfit.

Think of different ways to reward yourself at the end of your journey—and not with unhealthy food. Healthy rewards are incentives that mark achievements. I always want you to celebrate your small successes by telling your story at www.PeteThomas.com. You can also think of some ways to reward yourself when you've lost a few pounds or adopted a new Forever Habit to keep yourself motivated and on track. Maybe you can purchase some new exercise equipment, or take a friend golfing, or see that art exhibit you read about. Rewarding ourselves is going to be very important, because we will reach our goal by creating new habits that will help us Lose It Forever while applying those habits very aggressively to help us Lose It Fast.

KEY POINTS

- A great goal will keep you focused, encouraged, and motivated.
- A great weight loss goal needs to be S.M.A.R.T.: Specific, Measurable, Aggressive, Realistic, and Time-Based.
- Aggressive goals can be reached by creating Forever Habits to Lose It Forever, and then applying them aggressively to Lose It Fast.
- A Personal Success Statement will be more powerful if it is a personalized, positive, and present-tense affirmation.

CHAPTER 3 CHALLENGES

Write Down Your S.M.A.R.T. Goal

Now that you know how to make a S.M.A.R.T. Forever Goal, I want you to write it down in your LIF2 Success Journal. An example might be, "I want to lose 25 pounds in six months." We're not going to focus on this large goal, because we're going to be focused on forming healthy Forever

Habits. But these new habits will result in reaching this goal as we apply them aggressively in our lives. In other words, the Forever Goal (25 pounds, going down three dress sizes, or whatever) is the "what," and the Forever Habits are the "how."

Create Your Own Personal Success Statement

If possible, include your Lose It Forever goal in this statement. Be bold and confident in this statement by making it positive, personalized, and present tense. Show it to supportive friends or loved ones (we'll be talking about teammates in the next chapter) and get their opinion on it. Remember, we want it to be written as a personalized, positive, present-tense affirmation that preferably both rhymes and has some sort of emotional connection. I know it sounds complicated, but have fun with it. Write this statement down in your LIF2 Success Journal.

Take Several "Before" Photos

You can take these photos fully or partially clothed. I wanted to wear something revealing to take these shots. They are a great motivator, and cause for great celebration at the end of your journey. You can see one of my luscious "before" photos on the cover of this book, or go see others on my website. I keep them there as a motivator for myself and others who doubt their ability to lose a lot of weight.

Take several shots from the front and back and both sides. Take those pictures, put them in a sealed envelope, and give them to a few supportive people around you and tell them, "Hold on to these. One day there's going to be a new me, so I need you to store these in a safe place."

Put up the Photo of Your Goal Outfit

If you already own the outfit, put it in a place where you'll see it often. If you don't currently own it, then purchase it or download a picture from the Internet and post it someplace you will see it often.

Write Down Your Initial Weight and Measurements

Weigh yourself and write down your current weight. You're going to weigh yourself every week to track your progress, so you need a baseline weight. I want you to measure yourself, too. You'll measure yourself monthly. You can use the forms in LIF2 Success Journal to help you. If you can't download the LIF2 Success Journal, take the following measurements:

- Chest—at the widest portion
- Waist—where your waist bends
- Abdomen—across the belly button
- Hips—at the widest portion
- Thighs—at the widest portion of the right thigh, then multiply by two
- Arms—at the middle of the upper right arm, then multiply by two
- Total inches—add up the above six numbers to determine your total inches

Here are some tips for measuring yourself:

- Measure yourself once a month on the same day.
- Use a flexible measuring tape.
- When measuring, pull the tape moderately tight without stretching it.
- Measure naked if at all possible.
- Measure yourself in front of a mirror so that you can see if the tape is positioned correctly.
- Keep your muscles relaxed while measuring; do not flex your muscles.
- Get someone to measure you if it's helpful.

Create Another Top 10 List

Remember when you completed your Top 10 lists in Chapter 1? Now that you've learned about goal setting, I want you to rewrite your Top 5 Weight Loss Goals in a positive, present-tense fashion. Some of these might be social goals, such as "I attract attention from the opposite sex," or health-related goals, such as "I have normal blood pressure." Write this list in your journal, and be sure to include your plans for future events or milestones in life.

Review Your Goals Daily

Take time for yourself every day to review your goals. At least every morning, I want you to get up and repeat your Personal Success Statement. I want you to repeat those weight loss goals to yourself, making sure that you include the phrase "one Forever Habit at a time."

Write Down Your Reward System

How are you going to reward yourself when you've lost a few pounds or incorporated a Forever Habit into your life? As I said before, establishing some healthy rewards is going to be critical to staying motivated. Write those rewards down so that you can keep them in front of you.

"One of the key principles that Pete teaches is the importance of having supportive teammates—and for us, that means holding each other accountable for eating healthy food, tracking calories, and getting the exercise we need, whatever the time of day. It's been much easier for us to stick to our plan consistently because we feel responsible not only for our own decisions and results, but also for helping the other person be their best."

—MOLLY, LIF2 STUDENT

CHAPTER

GATHER A GREAT TEAM

HAVE YOU EVER BEEN IN TROUBLE WITH YOUR DIET? I DON'T MEAN like, "Oh, I ate that salad with real ranch dressing, so I need to run five more minutes on the treadmill." I mean real trouble, like, "If I eat this thing I know I shouldn't eat but I'm thinking about eating anyway, my whole diet is as good as gone." I have.

I got in trouble one day on *The Biggest Loser* Ranch, because I gave in to temptation. It was about six weeks into the second season of the show. I had left my life back in Michigan to concentrate on losing a lot of the 400-plus pounds I arrived with, and I was doing well, until this moment. Giving in to temptation is not hard to do at the ranch, because they put bad food all around the house. They even call them temptation foods. Now, keep in mind that there are cameras everywhere, because they are hoping to catch you sabotaging yourself. It makes for great TV if they can catch you getting up in the middle of the night and having a binge.

I came downstairs from my room one day and saw these colorful little things that had suddenly appeared in several small bowls in a display at the bottom of the stairs. I said, "What are these?" and reached in and tasted one. My knees buckled from the taste, as all at once this combination of chocolate and nuts just exploded in my mouth. I thought, "Oh, my goodness, this is amazing. What is this?" And so I reached in and I had a second, then a third, then a fourth, and a fifth. I ended up having a whole bowl of these things. And it got to me so badly that I thought that I was going to lose my mind if I didn't eat the next bowl and the next.

Before I completely destroyed myself, I yelled out to my buddy, "Mark! Where are you?" Mark immediately came down the stairs and asked me what was going on. I told him, "These things, they've got me." And so Mark, because he's a police officer, had to investigate. He reached in the jar and ate one. He said, "Oh, my goodness." His knees buckled as well.

Mark told me, "Pete, these are chocolate Jordan almonds. They're famous at weddings." Well, I grew up in the inner city of Detroit, so I'd never tasted a chocolate Jordan almond before. But I had been missing chocolate for quite a few weeks. I knew I was close to the edge.

We both knew we had to get these "hell-nuts" out of the house if we were going to succeed. They were bad news. We immediately cleared out all the chocolate Jordan almonds from every location in the house and put them in the trash. The art department was responsible for setting up the pretty food decorations for television, and they were in a tizzy because we had taken down all of that week's decorations. But we knew it was either them or us.

We dumped all the chocolate-covered almonds in the trash container by the laundry room. Problem solved, right?

Wrong! If you are a compulsive eater like me, you can predict the dilemma that was about to take place. The laundry room is a very important place on a workout show. We worked out three to four hours a day and washed clothes a couple of times a day. I walked in and out of the laundry room all the time.

That particular day I went in and out about three or four times. And every time I walked by that trash can, those chocolate Jordan almonds would whisper to me, "Pete, eat me. Pete, eat me." And at some point I just could not resist. I knew there were no cameras in that location, so I looked around to make sure no one was watching. The coast was clear, so I reached into the trash and pulled out some of the almonds.

I knew that I was in a bad spot. I felt myself losing it. I remember thinking, "I am going to get kicked off *The Biggest Loser* for eating out of a garbage can!" So I called Mark again. We had to come up with a "permanent" solution. He and I ended up pouring liquid laundry detergent all over those chocolate Jordan almonds that were already in the trash can.

I tell this story to demonstrate the importance of one enormous factor in the weight loss equation—a factor many people overlook.

THE BIGGEST LOSER "SECRET SAUCE"

Why had I quit my diets in the past and gained back all the weight that I had lost? There are a variety of reasons, but one of the most important is also the most overlooked. It's so simple that people miss it in their search for some complicated hormonal or genetic answer. What was I lacking in my quest for better health? Was it a magic pill or special workout or something to sprinkle on my food? It was none of the above. What was I, like so many other people, lacking?

A team.

That's right. A team. While I had committed to fighting my "enemy" for myself, I knew I could not win the battle by myself.

Now, I know what you may be thinking, and it's true—a team by itself did not cause me to lose weight. I had to address issues in my mind, alter my diet, and create new exercise habits. But I truly believe the lack of a team may be the "make or break" element that keeps us on the program or causes us to get discouraged and quit. It was for me.

There have been a lot of articles written on *The Biggest Loser* weight loss approach. A lot of critics have commented on the contestants' dieting habits and our workout regimens, as well as the presence of professional trainers, even though they have never stepped foot on the ranch and are hardly experts from viewing a few episodes. But most of these people overlook the most potent factor that the show brings to its contestants—

its "secret sauce," if you will. That factor is a strong, supportive, twenty-four-hour-a-day team environment among the contestants.

I experienced this sense of being part of a team for the first time in my life while I was on *The Biggest Loser* Ranch. I've already told you a little bit about my background, how I grew up transient as a child because my mother suffered from mental illness and was very unstable. As a result, I moved constantly from city to city and state to state. Eventually I was taken away and put into the foster care system. Because I was changing locations so much, I never joined a sports team or stayed in any one school very long. So I didn't know how powerful a motivator a team could be until I showed up at the ranch.

BATTLE OF THE SEXES

I'll never forget that very first morning we contestants showed up at *The Biggest Loser* Ranch. We had been packed into these white fifteen-passenger vans in the middle of the night and driven out to Hummingbird Ranch in Simi Valley, California, where we would be filming the show.

We stumbled out of the vans while it was still dark and we began to shoot hours of footage as day broke while walking up and down the hills that made up the driveway of the ranch. Since we had not eaten breakfast, we were hungry and tired, so naturally we started to complain. Mostly about being hungry and tired. You don't want to make a herd of chubbies hungry and tired—that's a bad combination.

But our producer was not sympathetic to our complaining. Rather, he told us to suck it up, that we eventually would be fed and that we were being given a once-in-a-lifetime opportunity to regain our lives. We all wanted to eat him! But good news was to follow, as we were soon given our first taste of the "team" nature of the show that season. After we had finally made it up that awful hill several times, the host revealed that our teams would be the most basic and competitive of all: men versus women. The camaraderie of this arrangement was not only crucial to my success but provided great drama for viewers of the show. We encouraged each other toward our personal goals, of course, but we also genuinely wanted to beat the other team!

Prior to this moment I had no idea how powerful a team could be when you're trying to do something as critical as losing weight. There is no way I can overstate this—you cannot lose weight alone. This lifestyle change you are contemplating is not like deciding whether or not a new outfit of clothes looks good on you. It's a little more important than that. And yet most of us would be more likely to seek help or guidance about a new outfit than we would about weight loss. We would discuss it with our best friend or spouse, look at a catalog to see how the models look in the outfit, or post a picture on Facebook and ask for comments. We would include all these different people in our process. But when it comes to weight loss, many of us want to do it alone.

Weight loss is one of those things that people think, "Oh, I can do this on my own." Dumb, dumb, dumb. Weight loss is not something you're going to be successful at on your own. Now, you may be asking, "Why do I need a team?" A team is important for a lot of reasons. But here are the two main ones: accountability and encouragement.

TEAMWORK MAKES THE DREAM WORK, OR HOW TO DEVELOP DISCIPLINE

Accountability is one of the major reasons to gather a great team. We can develop self-discipline by allowing others to keep us honest in the decisions we are making. Our goal in allowing someone to hold us accountable is so that, eventually, self-discipline will take hold to the point where we no longer need the external discipline of someone checking up on us. But accountability from others is essential, especially at the beginning of our weight loss journey.

Here are four groups of people we should allow to hold us accountable. I had come up with these four groups in my own research; then I read an article by fitness guru and author Tom Venuto, who mentioned them in a nice succinct way, although in a different order. I like to think of them as a pyramid:

1. The public
   The public can be brutal! Or very encouraging and motivating. Think of the relationship that sports teams have with their schools. Going

"public" can help us move toward our goals because of this positive and negative motivation. Go public with your goals and work hard to not let the public down! Millions of viewers each week provided this to us contestants on *The Biggest Loser*. But you don't need to be on TV; you can use social media to make your goals public—write a blog about committing to weight loss for good; post your goals on Facebook and ask people to help you; write a Twitter post that says, "I am starting my LIF2 journey—who is with me or been there?" or "One more LIF2 Forever Habit in place." There are lots of ways to let the public encourage you or hold you accountable, even if you're not involved with social media. You could write a letter to family members, or simply make an announcement at a social gathering. Just put your goals out there!

2. A large group or team

Groups of like-minded individuals with similar goals can spark energy into our goals and keep us on target. Teams do great things together and are a great source of accountability. The "Guys" team on *The Biggest Loser* fulfilled this layer of accountability for me. Maybe you have a team of people at work who are all trying to lose weight, or a group of your friends who can all go through this book together. Take advantage of the extended LIF2 team by posting comments at the LIF2 Facebook page, then share it with your other social media sites. There is going to be some natural overlap between our "public" accountability and our "team" accountability. In fact, making our goals public—at work for instance—might help us find a smaller team of like-minded people. It takes effort to put together a team, but nothing will help you more in the long run.

3. A trainer, mentor, or teammate

This is typically that one other person who can relate to us in an intimate one-on-one fashion. One person can typically develop a stronger individual connection and speak to us in ways that larger groups can't. They can also challenge us face-to-face to accomplish our goals. Jillian Michaels was this to me, and I am this to many others. They should check in with you frequently to make sure you're meeting your goals and making progress. You can reach out to them for help whenever you're having a tough time to get back on track. This person could be a spouse or a friend if they can "hold your feet to the fire."

But if this person is not likely to be tough on you, it might be a good idea to find someone outside your circle of influence.

4. Yourself: self-mastery, self-control, self-discipline

You've made it! You set individual goals on your own. You track progress on your own. You put in extra work on your own. You do it not because someone has told you to do it, but because it matters to you alone. You are your own best teammate. You are accountable to yourself and have developed discipline—in at least one area of life. Finally, over seven years after leaving *The Biggest Loser,* I can say that I am self-disciplined in the area of my nutrition and exercise.

THE REASON I LIKE to view these groups as a pyramid is because the first three groups (the public, a team, and a coach) work to help us develop self-discipline because they help impose external discipline upon us. External discipline is imposed until we develop strong internal discipline.

An example of this is when parents tell their children to brush their teeth and then follow up this simple activity for years—helped by periodic stern warnings from the dentist—until it becomes second nature in the child. By the same token the public, a team, or a trainer can help put external pressure upon us to accomplish our goals until internal discipline takes over.

To develop self-mastery, you need all the other collaborators, all the other teammates. Great teammates lead to great accomplishments. We'll discuss how to find your teammates and build your team for success later this chapter.

TRUE ACCOUNTABILITY

I read a blog post by a business consultant named Ann Evanston about the nature of accountability that I really like. I will share it with you because accountability can be painful, but it's important to get this part right. Her words may sound harsh, but let's be honest—sometimes we need someone harsh to keep us honest.

What does being in an accountability group or having an accountability partner mean to you? For me it means someone who holds me accountable to a commitment I made. Simple enough. If I am asked to hold you accountable, that means that I am not there to rally behind when you fail. To sympathize with you when you did not make your commitment. I'm not there to support the excuse you have or the lie you tell yourself as to why you did not keep your commitment.

I am there to question why. To push you to get back on track. To challenge the excuses you might be telling yourself. I will be the accountability you will HATE at times. The accountability that calls you on your excuses and lies, and challenges you to get real with yourself. I will be the accountability that pisses you off, makes you mad, maybe even cry at times.

It will be accountability that you deserve. Because you are worth the commitment you made to yourself. To who you are. To the success you want to have.

We will put these concepts into action at the end of the chapter when we write down some practical steps to assure ourselves of accountability.

TRUE ENCOURAGEMENT

Encouragement is just as important as accountability. Being on *The Biggest Loser* was like being in a family. The crew, the people that are filming the show behind the scenes, they want you to do well. The medical staff, the trainers, the producers, they're all part of the team. And you've got your teammates, the other contestants, who understand the struggles that you're going through like no one else, and they want you to do well.

Sometimes all it takes is an understanding word to keep you going when the journey gets hard. We had a relay race challenge on the show that involved carrying small weighted medicine balls through a series of train cars. I don't know how much they weighed, but it felt like we were carrying bags of cement through the boxcars. It was incredibly hard. I had carried this thing as far as I could go—I was sure I could not go another step. At that moment, one of the camera operators—who are not supposed to be seen or heard—said to me, "Good job. You're doing great, Pete!" Those encouraging words allowed me to keep pushing through the pain and anguish. Kind words can do that—they are like wind in your sails when you feel like giving up. So do your best to surround yourself with people who will offer those kind words during hard times.

THE SOCIAL INFLUENCE OF A TEAM

I've already told you why I believe teams are important for weight loss and how they helped me personally lose weight and keep it off forever. Several recent studies have been done that show that extended social networks affect our weight and our health. Birds of a feather flock together. If you are overweight you tend to have the same types of overweight friends and romantic interests. And health-conscious people tend to have friends who are also health-conscious. What I have personally learned is that I can change the birds I flock together with and have an impact on all of the other birds around me.

BUILDING YOUR TEAM

I am often asked, "How many teammates do I need?" My answer is, the more the merrier! You will encounter many obstacles on your path to better health, so you need a wide variety of teammates to support you on your journey.

We will find these teammates all around us: family members, friends, coworkers, members of your spiritual community, fellow exercisers at the gym; we can even find teammates online. So how should we look for teammates?

First, we can evaluate the people closest to us. We need to make a list of all the people around us and mark whether they are positive, negative, or neutral about our weight loss goals. This means, of course, that we are going to have to tell them about our goals. Telling people will let us know right away whether they are going to be supportive or not based on their reactions. You want to build your team only with people who are positive and supportive of your weight loss goals.

TEAM MEMBERS

Your team members probably are going to fall into one of the two categories I talked about earlier.

ACCOUNTABILITY TEAMMATES:

- Medical teammates
- Workout teammates
- Coaches and trainers
- Food teammates
- S.W.A.T. teammates

ENCOURAGEMENT TEAMMATES:

- Shoulder teammates
- Spiritual teammates
- Work teammates
- Online teammates

Accountability Teammates

First and foremost, you need to consult your physician—your main medical teammate—before you pursue any new diet or exercise regimen. Your medical teammates will be important at the beginning, as they give you permission to exert yourself, but they will also be important as you exercise because you will experience some aches and pains. We also need to train our medical teammates concerning our goals.

I say this because quite often when you see your doctor about some ache brought on by exercise, your doctor is going to say, "Well, stop doing what you're doing and it won't hurt anymore." That is really unacceptable if you are going to become healthy long-term.

I had to train my own doctor. A few years ago I hurt my ankle playing basketball. After a thorough exam and X-rays, my doctor said, "Pete, it looks like you've got torn ligaments in your ankle." He went on to say that I had two options. He said, "One, we can do surgery. Or you can let the ankle heal, since 90 percent of torn ankle ligaments heal on their own." I wanted to let my torn ligaments heal, but I wasn't willing to take a step back in my weight loss goals while that was happening. Because I've trained my doctor, he knows that I'm not going to stop exercising or stop working out. We have a great relationship. That comes part and parcel with training your physician.

When I told him it only hurt when I ran outdoors, he recommended that I keep running but stay indoors. So over the course of that year I was able to stay physically fit because I ran indoors. I put a lot of time on the treadmill and the StairMaster, which provide more of a cushion for your joints, and it worked out fine—I healed up without a problem. Now, if you really are too injured to run, your doctor will let you know. If that's the case, don't lose your exercising habit. If you're too injured to do a certain activity, do another exercise in its place. Take a swimming class. Jump on a bike. Taking time off may not be necessary; just change your activity.

Workout Teammates

Of course we will need workout teammates. Someone who will go with us to the gym and sweat with us, or someone who will come over and exercise to a DVD right beside us. Loafing is incredibly easy if we don't have a steady workout partner. Our bodies do not want to work as hard as we need them to, and our mind is not always going to be our friend. We need someone to keep us exercising.

When it comes to working out, we need three types of teammates, which I'll explain more below.

- We need teammates who are more advanced so they can inspire us to improve.
- We need teammates who are at our level so they can keep us accountable.
- We need teammates who are not yet at our level so that we can "reach out" and cement our weight loss goals.

I think it's very important to have someone who is more experienced and knowledgeable than you at a particular thing, who really can show you how to eat correctly and how to work out correctly. Coaches and trainers can be very helpful when it comes to learning to work out more effectively as well. I am a coach to the students in my boot camp, and having me around makes them work a little harder. People with that kind of authority instill a healthy fear—you don't want to disappoint your coach or trainer, so you might push a little bit harder when you feel like quitting.

You also need someone *at* your level, someone right around where you are. Maybe this is the teammate that you take to the gym and work out with. He or she needs to be at the same point in the weight loss journey as you so they can keep you working as hard as you can. It's like studying a subject in college—two students working together can relate to and encourage each other. I had many workout partners on *The Biggest Loser*, but I especially enjoyed working out with my fellow contestant Mark. He helped push me to match him, and I needed that. In this case, peer pressure was a good thing.

You may find it strange, but I believe we also need to have someone who's a little behind us—kind of a mentee—that we can bring along on our journey. That's because as we learn about health and wellness and nutrition and exercise, these things will become even more solidified in our minds as we turn around and touch others. This has certainly been true for me as I've taught students how to lose weight permanently in my classes.

Food Teammates

We will also need food teammates. We all need someone to hold us accountable when it comes to the food we're eating. After more than seven successful years off the ranch, I still need someone who is willing to look over my food journals and food logs or simply ask me what I'm consuming. We need food teammates who are close enough that they can check what we're eating on a weekly basis. This can be a family member, a friend, or a coworker—someone who sees us eat regularly. To be effective, however, we need to be completely honest about what we're eating.

When I go out to a restaurant with my food teammates, I've given them permission to ask me, "Pete, is that what you should be eating, or can you eat something just a little bit better?" Those words may irk you at first, but they can save you from heartache later.

S.W.A.T. Teammates

S.W.A.T. teams come into a hostile environment and rescue hostages. Everyone needs a S.W.A.T. teammate when they are dieting—someone who will help us say "No!" when we are being held hostage by some nasty food. This person can be someone who lives with you or someone you can call when you're in trouble. A S.W.A.T. teammate is a person of action who is not afraid to throw something in the trash if it is hindering your progress. Mark was this teammate for me at *The Biggest Loser* Ranch. I've already told you a story about how he helped keep me on the straight and narrow with those Jordan almonds.

Encouragement Teammates

During our weight loss journey, we will get down emotionally from time to time. That's why we need teammates who encourage us. Sometimes we need what I call a shoulder teammate. That is the person who gives us a shoulder to cry on, who will hear us out when we say, "Life is really tough right now. Help me get through."

Dr. Jeffrey Levine fulfilled this role for me at *The Biggest Loser* Ranch. Despite his physical limitations—he started out with some pretty severe ankle problems—Dr. Jeff was an awesome teammate. Because he and I were closer in terms of ability, we were often paired together to work out. So he and I spent loads of time together, and everything about him was a support to me.

I remember one particular time on the ranch, six or seven weeks into the show, I was tired of the entire experience. Not just tired of the intense workout schedule, but sick of everybody around me.

That particular night was very important, because it was the night before a weigh-in. We were in the gym and the women's team started complaining about me sweating and grunting or some such silly thing, and I decided, "You know what? I've had it. I'm through." Spending seven weeks looking at the same fourteen fat people (myself included) 24/7 will drive you absolutely bonkers! I left the gym immediately and went out back to the patio. I just sat down and started sulking. I wanted to go home right then and there.

Soon after that, Dr. Jeff came into the gym and looked around. He didn't find me. So being the great teammate that he is, he decided to go find his buddy. He completely ditched his workout to find me. Now, remember, we're on a workout show. You do not ditch a workout. That's like a chef on a cooking show saying, "Oh, never mind. Forget it. I'm just going out for fast food. I'm not cooking." Ditching a workout on a weight loss show just does not happen.

But that is why Dr. Jeff was such a special teammate. He found me, and we sat for hours just talking about family and the things that we missed, as well as all the things that we were going to do back home as we continued on this weight loss journey. He did more than give me a shoulder to cry on. He inspired me. He pushed me. He encouraged me.

Later that night, around two in the morning, I went back into the gym to finish my final hard hour of intense exercise. That was pivotal for me, because that particular week I lost more weight than the entire girls' team put together. That weight loss helped to save us from elimination, as another one of my teammates did not do well that week.

Spiritual Teammate

Maybe you would enjoy working out four hours a day weighing over 400 pounds, but I didn't! My confidence was at an all-time low during those first few weeks at *The Biggest Loser* Ranch. The weight was coming off slowly, my trainer threatened to take my life each and every day, and I was not permitted any contact with the outside world or my loved ones.

That's why my roommate, Seth, was literally a "godsend." At the end of every day, after literally trying to work my tail off, I would stumble into the room and collapse onto this twin bed made for someone half my size. As my body began to recover, all these emanations would start to come from my body, from all parts of my body. Don't pretend you don't know what I'm talking about. Poor Seth—these little noises would wake him up in the middle of the night. But he never held the lack of sleep against me.

On the contrary, Seth made himself a wonderful spiritual partner. Every night we would pray for our loved ones back home, and we would pray for each other as well. He was a great comfort to me, because he would remind me every night, "Okay, Pete, let's pray." I certainly needed the prayers back then, and I still do.

Because some of our weight struggles are rooted in childhood and how we were raised, we may need a spiritual teammate to help us deal with them. As we've discussed, the battle to lose weight occurs first in the mind, so we need a spiritual teammate to keep us grounded. Maybe the person you live with is not a supportive spiritual teammate. You may need a pastor, a prayer partner from your spiritual community, or a trained therapist who can help you through some of these things.

Work Teammates

For those of us who work outside the home, we will need workplace teammates. These coworkers are critical, because most people spend a majority of their time at work. You probably already know that there are many ways to lose focus on your health goals when you're at work. The power lunches. The meeting donuts. The snack cravings.

We need workplace teammates who will encourage us to eat healthy snacks and meals while we're away from home. Sometimes these workplace teammates can provide "competition" to make the weight loss process more interesting. Maybe you have coworkers who are also losing weight. Having a friendly contest is a great motivator. I have spoken at many companies who are kicking off weight loss competitions. They really work. Your company may already have such a contest going. If you need help starting one, contact me. We've got resources to help.

So having a workplace teammate—preferably someone who's following one of my weight loss programs along with you—is going to be great for you. If you don't have a workplace teammate right now, encourage a colleague to get a copy of *Lose It Fast, Lose It Forever* and work through it together.

Online Teammates

To really lose weight consistently, we may need online teammates. The neat thing about the Internet is that we can get support from people who are at the same place in our weight loss journey but who live half a continent away. These are people with whom we can communicate regularly. Shooting these teammates a quick e-mail to let them know how we're doing will help us stay the course. It's all part of that regular accountability that is so important.

Remember that there is a certain amount of anonymity that you can maintain in an online relationship, whether it be in one of the forums or on a social site. There are pros and cons to a "faceless" relationship like that. There's typically a certain amount of acceptance, which can be good in your struggle to gain back your health. The negative side of that is that someone online can be completely accepting of every behavior we engage in, because they aren't always aware of what we're actually doing. They're not in our face, challenging our decisions. While that can be appealing, it may not be the best thing for us. Just be careful in your virtual relationships, that you exploit the good and avoid the bad.

CHOOSING THE RIGHT TEAMMATES

A word of warning: Choosing teammates who are saboteurs rather than supporters can be detrimental to your health. So it's important that you figure out how to select the right partners for the journey. One of the most important things you can do is analyze your family and friends and assess whether or not they're positive teammates. I mentioned this earlier when I told you to tell everyone about your weight loss goals so you can see their reactions. You'll have to judge them on the following qualities.

Temperament

Not everyone around you is going to make a good teammate. I had a teammate on *The Biggest Loser* Ranch who was a negative influence for me. He was extremely funny and a riot to hang out with, but he balked when it came to Jillian and her methods. It got to the point where Jillian would get angry at the rest of us because we would laugh at the jokes he told at her expense and we would still include him at dinner, even though he was following his own workout regimen and not the workouts Jillian designed. She felt like it was a slap in her face because she believed that everybody should be on board with what we were trying to do as a group. Ultimately we had to agree with her. When it came time to vote someone off the ranch, we voted this guy off because he didn't have the right type of personality for our success. You need to find teammates who will support your goals, not sabotage them.

Availability

Needless to say, availability is key. Sometimes potentially good teammates don't work out because they're never around when we need them. If they have completely opposite work schedules to ours or a lot of family commitments, that could be a real issue when we need help.

Teammates should be nearby, especially if you're going to go work out with them. If your teammate is going to meet you at the track or the gym or in front of a workout DVD on a regular basis, it needs to be convenient for both of you.

Strengths and Weaknesses

What are the strengths or weaknesses of your teammates? Do they complement your own strengths? If your strength is working out but your weakness is eating, you may want to consider having a teammate whose weakness is working out but whose strength is eating. This way, you can both help each other reach your goals.

That was the way it was with Matt and me on *The Biggest Loser*. Matt, the eventual grand prize winner in our season, always worked out really, really hard. I never reached Matt's workout level, partially due to the fact that he was younger and had been a successful collegiate athlete. He always pushed himself as hard as possible. He was amazing to watch. Yet at times he was so self-disciplined that he was often a loner when it came to the gym. I still looked to him for inspiration, though. I have tried to follow his example on the show and help others in that same way.

TEACH OR TERMINATE

You may have to deal with a thorny issue regarding your teammates. What do you do if a teammate is unsupportive? I believe that you have two options. You've got to either teach them or you've got to terminate them. Once we share our goals with teammates, they need to get with the program—our program.

Let's be honest. There are certain people who will follow their instinct or habits, without any thought as to how it's affecting you. In many ways, the situation of a compulsive eater is similar to that of an alcoholic. An alcoholic will have friends whose natural proclivity is to go out to the bar on Friday night and drink a lot. That's a problem if you're an alcoholic.

For those of us who are overweight, our struggle is eating poorly or eating without restraint. Inevitably you'll have teammates who, when they go out to eat or when they go out to have fun, will eat unhealthy foods without really thinking about it. You can do a couple of things. You can suggest, "Hey, could we go someplace different?" Or "Could you try to change what you eat when we're together?" They need to be taught how to help you. At some point, hopefully, they'll get it. What you want to do is recommend the same thing over and over: "Hey, can we go someplace different and eat, someplace that has some healthy options?" Better yet, suggest an activity that doesn't include eating, like going for a walk or attending a concert. You want to try to influence them.

I have some good friends who for years have been including me at different events at their house. So when I got back from the show I said to them, "You know, I never noticed it before the show, but I see that you don't have any diet pop, veggies, or salad." Of course, they're much smaller than I was and they've never had to think about any of that. And they said, "No, we're sorry." So I said, "Okay." I still hung out, but I didn't really eat much.

The next time they invited me over, the conversation went like this.

"Hey, you guys still don't have any salad or diet pop?"

"No, we forgot."

"Okay. I'll see you later."

"Hey, where are you going?"

"Somewhere else. You don't have anything that I can eat. I asked for it last time and you haven't made any changes."

"Oh. Well, can you just stay this time?"

"No. I'll see you later."

The next time they called, they said, "Pete, can you come to our family event? By the way, we've got some diet pop, we've got some salad, we've got some baked chicken and things that you like."

Now, it's very interesting what started happening. At different social events, even church events that typically featured high-calorie "comfort" foods, once the healthier options were made available—like serving water instead of soda pop—those healthier options were the first things to go.

A lot of times we serve bad foods just out of habit, not realizing that people probably would choose the healthier options if they were available.

My point is, we can teach people. We can teach our teammates, friends, and loved ones that we want healthier options or we're not coming over. You might want to follow the suggestions I give in Chapter 9 for bringing your own food to a party if your loved ones are slow to understand, but our goal is to teach people. Most people will get it. If they don't, we'll have to terminate those relationships. Like we tell our children, that's when we realize that they weren't friends to begin with. Of course, people in your family are different; if they are not supportive, we have to really work on the teaching part because we can't just walk away from them. But we may have to terminate other social relationships. When I use the word "terminate," don't get me wrong, I don't mean that in the organized crime sense—I just mean you need to move on to another more beneficial, healthier relationship.

SIGNED CONTRACT

One of the key things that I want you to consider is asking your teammates to sign a contract with you, stating they will support you and will not sabotage you. This is especially important to do with your spouse or significant other. Although you're going to take complete personal ownership of your own weight loss, you need support. You need to know that your closest relationships are going to help, not hinder, your journey to health. Use the following short contract as an example (or you can download a copy at www.PeteThomas.com) to let them know you are serious:

I, _____, promise to support _____ in his/her goal of becoming healthier by changing one Forever Habit at a time. I will not keep dangerous foods in the house or eat tempting foods in front of her/him except by mutual agreement. I promise to help him/her by being an encouraging and accountable partner. I will try never to be negative or say the goal is impossible. I am dedicated to his/her success!

_____ (Sign and date)

Now, HOPEFULLY, they'll have to help you, because you've got their signature on a contract! And believe me, we need all the help we can get to reach our goal.

COMMUNICATING WITH YOUR TEAM

Never be shy about asking for help. Your life may literally depend on being successful in this venture. Our teammates can do lots of things to help us get our health back. They can help us shop for food. Our team can even help us prepare food. They can take over some of our chores to free up time to exercise. They can watch the children for a few hours. They can plan activities that don't include eating. They can really help make this whole experience fun and interesting.

So what I want you to do is look at the following list of how your team can help you reach your goals. Decide which items on the list are applicable and who might be able to help with them. In the Challenges section, you are going to fill out a chart assigning specific duties to your team. You will give them to your teammates so they can know exactly what areas you need help with. And if you need something, ask!

Our teammates can help us reach our goals by helping us in many ways, including shopping for us, encouraging us to cook healthy new foods, reminding us of our goals, walking with us, and taking on some of our chores to free up time for exercising. I have provided a chart with a long list of jobs your teammates can take on in the Challenges section of this chapter. Also on the chart is a blank space beside each job so that you can assign it to someone on your team.

GATHER YOUR TEAM

Studies show, and *The Biggest Loser* has demonstrated, that having a supportive team around you can be that one added factor that makes you successful at pursuing a healthier life. So don't try to do this on your own. Follow the steps in this chapter and build a healthy team around you, and then get going on building a healthy life, one Forever Habit at a time. As you succeed, touch an online teammate by telling your story at www.PeteThomas.com.

As you continue down the road to healthier living, do not be afraid to rearrange your team. If you've watched *The Biggest Loser,* you know that one of the twists is rearranging teams or switching trainers. One of the reasons we get complacent is because we stick with the same team beyond the point where they're actually helping. At certain times you may need to change your trainer, or change your workout partner, or any other partner who is no longer helping you move forward.

KEY POINTS

- A great team, supplying both accountability and encouragement, could be the make-or-break element in your weight loss success.
- Effective accountability is found on four levels: the public, a team, a coach, and finally to yourself.
- If a teammate is unsupportive, you've got to either teach or terminate that person.
- Don't be afraid to ask for help!

CHAPTER 4 CHALLENGES

Write Down Your Accountability

List some ways you can be accountable according to the four layers of accountability. For example, for the first layer, perhaps you could post your weight loss goals on a website for everybody to view. For the second layer, could you form a competition at work for people who want to lose weight? For the third layer, list a mentor or team member who could hold you accountable. And finally, how could you hold yourself to your goals? Making a chart like the following might be helpful.

Layer of Accountability	How can I take advantage?
#1: The public	
#2: Team or group	
#3: Coach, trainer, mentor, or teammate	
#4: Self	

Announce Your Intention to Lose Weight

Now you're going public. Go to all of your friends and family and tell them about your new goal. You should have made some specific goals after reading the last chapter. Now I want you to tell the people around you that you are making a serious effort to lose some weight. Tell them the long-term goal, and then mention that you're going to lose it by changing one Forever Habit at a time.

We do that for one main reason. We need to mark them—either they're supporters or they're saboteurs. We want to note those people who are saboteurs on the list right away. We're not going to tell them a lot in the future about our weight loss goals and we're not going to depend on them for emotional support. You can record people's attitudes in your journal to keep track, if necessary.

Build a Supportive Team

I want you to make a list of all your relationships and evaluate them based on the qualities I've mentioned in the chart below. You can find this chart on my website, www.PeteThomas.com, or simply create one like it. Then choose some teammates. The next action step will help with that, because you'll know who's going to be supportive and who isn't.

BUILDING A SUPPORT TEAM

Think about relationships—spouse, partner, roommates, children, mother, father, grandmothers, grandfathers, aunts, uncles, friends, work friends, coaches, and others.

Name and relationship	Positive Attitudes, words, and actions	Negative Attitudes, words, and actions	Neutral Attitudes, words, and actions
Pete Thomas (coach)	X		

Assign Roles to Your Teammates

We have discussed the importance of letting our team help us as we take this weight loss journey. Look at the list of how our teammates can help us and assign roles and jobs to specific teammates. You can download this list from my website or make your own. Make several copies and give them to members of your team. Don't forget to communicate with them about their role in making you successful!

Role of Teammate	Name of Teammate
• Shop for food	
• Prepare food	
• Help me look for new healthy foods	
• Encourage me to taste and cook healthy new foods	
• Serve low-fat/calorie meals	
• Eat low-fat/calorie meals with me	
• Keep high-fat/calorie food out of sight	
• Keep healthy foods in sight	
• Plan the meal for me	
• Plate the meal for me	
• Put food away as soon as meal is plated	
• Don't offer me second helpings	
• Clear the table and dishes	
• Don't put the serving bowl on the table	
• Put food away as soon as meal is over	
• Don't offer me bad food options	
• Don't eat bad food options in front of me	
• Take over some chores to free up time	
• Help me find time for activities	
• Help me plan activities that don't include eating	
• Suggest activities that are active	
• Walk with me	
• Exercise with me	
• Buy healthy-themed gifts	
• Help me make it fun and interesting	
• Remind me of my goals	
• Don't make it easy for me to fail	
• Don't give in if I want to cheat	
• Praise my efforts	

FOREVER FUNDAMENTALS— STEP ONE CHECKLIST

AFTER READING STEP ONE: YOUR POWER, YOU SHOULD HAVE A MUCH better understanding about our relationship with food and how you got to the place where you are. You should have a solid commitment to taking this weight loss journey, which starts with setting aside time for yourself. You have set some great S.M.A.R.T. goals to keep your motivation strong, and gathered a great team to encourage you and hold you accountable. You should have begun a food journal to track what goes into your mouth and initiated some light exercise. You should have formed, or be in the process of forming, the following Forever Habits as you seek to truly Master Your Mind. Make note of the habits that you need to work on and try to come up with a plan to start implementing them.

STEP 1: YOUR POWER, FOREVER HABITS

- Write down your feelings about eating in your LIF2 Success Journal.
- Keep a record of what you eat in your LIF2 Success Journal.
- Review your Personal Power Goals.
- Put "me time" on your calendar and keep the appointment every day.
- Find a non-eating way to de-stress.
- Articulate your S.M.A.R.T. goal.
- Recite your Personal Success Statement.
- Weigh yourself on a regular basis.
- Build a good support team.
- Revise your team as new challenges arise.
- Communicate regularly with your teammates about your progress or needs.
- Make sure you have accountability in place and communicate regularly with your team.
- Be a good, involved teammate for someone else trying to Lose It Forever.

With these Forever Habits in place, or in the process of being formed within us, it is time to move with confidence to Step 2: Your Plan.

STEP TWO

YOUR PLAN

"I have tried different variations of losing weight in the past—Weight Watchers, South Beach, Atkins, and I would lose weight with each, but it always came back. The biggest problem I found with those diets was that they would tell you what you could or couldn't eat, but you didn't have the knowledge to make smart decisions. I loved that LIF2 gave me all the tools and knowledge I need to help me make better choices on my own. To date, I've lost about 65 pounds and I have become a much more physically fit person. My doctor was amazed at the progress I made in one year. It is an awesome feeling!"

—JESSICA, LIF2 STUDENT

CHAPTER

MANAGE YOUR MOUTH

WHAT DO YOU LIKE TO DO ON FRIDAY NIGHT? YOU'VE HAD A LONG workweek and you're tired. You need to relax somehow. Some people like to drink or party on Friday nights. I'm not really into that, so what do I do? Well, now I engage in healthy activities—but before I went on *The Biggest Loser,* I liked to eat. Before I went on the show, I would literally drug myself with food. I ate a lot—and it was killing me very slowly. I'll let you in on a typical pre–*Biggest Loser* Friday night.

Because I had not mastered my mind, I would want to reward myself with food. I would start by going to the Outback Steakhouse near my house. The Old Pete was especially fond of the cheese fries they served as an appetizer. And when I sat down to eat those cheese fries, the people around me soon figured out that those were *my* fries. I was not sharing these with anyone else. You can't have them. Back up. Don't even look at my cheese fries. I ate those all by myself. This appetizer would be followed by a typical steakhouse meal, including dessert.

Then after the steakhouse, I went out to the movies. When I got there, I ordered a large, hot-buttered movie popcorn. Now, I couldn't just walk up to the counter and order a large, hot-buttered movie popcorn. I had to specialize the order Pete Thomas style. So I would tell the little sixteen-year-old who was serving me, "This is what I want you to do. Put in twelve kernels and stop. Add some butter right there. Now put in twelve more kernels, stop, and add some butter right there. Twelve more kernels, stop, and add some butter right there. Repeat that eight to ten times, and then at the end of that bucket being filled, we've got the perfect popcorn." I ate this, as well as a box or two of candy, every Friday night at the movies.

Pop quiz: Do you think I was gaining or losing weight on a typical Friday night? Even more basic: Was this type of eating good or bad for me? Inherently it was bad. But why? No one had ever told me why! That's because no one ever told me what I am about to explain to you.

FILL 'ER UP

I mentioned this briefly in the Introduction, but it bears repeating: In our educational system the way most people learn is through *systematic education*. We learn our alphabet before we learn about nouns and verbs and finally sentences. Our ABCs are the lowest common denominator, but we must learn these first if we're going to communicate effectively.

When it comes to nutrition education, we don't do this. We learn more complex things first, like salt and fat and carbs and recommended daily allowances—and very few people ever learn their nutritional ABCs. We complicate the discussion even further with points, serving sizes, "natural foods," and other confusing terms.

PETE'S BASIC NUTRITION INFORMATION EQUATION

- Humans require fuel for energy to function.
- Energy for humans comes from food.

- The energy in food is measured in calories (technically kilocalories, or kcals—each calorie we count actually contains one thousand units of energy).
- The body uses a certain number of calories for energy every day. Extra calories are stored as fat for days when the body may not receive the number of calories it needs to function.
- Calories consumed determines weight gain or loss.

Calories are the lowest common denominator in the energy equation. Calories in food come from fats, carbs, and proteins (these are called macronutrients). So the following formula is as basic as it gets when it comes to losing weight.

WEIGHT LOSS 101
1. Lose weight = Reduce calories
2. Reduce calories = Reduce fats, carbs, and proteins (macronutrients)
3. Lose weight further = Reduce calories and carb ratio (more about this in the next chapter)

Food is fuel—that's all it is. Food is fuel for the body, just like gasoline is fuel for the automobile. Fortunately, we actually get to enjoy the fuel that we consume. The problem comes when we enjoy it a little too much, when we focus so much on the enjoyment part that we forget about the providing energy part.

A calorie is simply a unit of energy that comes from the food you eat. We are like automobiles in our need for fuel. We need so many calories a day to function, and that number depends on your gender, your size, and your activity level.

You may be asking, "Why does my body need fuel?" Simple. All our organs require energy to keep us alive. Basal life processes like respiration (breathing), blood circulation, the beating of our hearts, and using our muscles all require energy. Believe it or not, about 70 percent of a human's total energy expenditure is due to these processes within the organs of the body.

Another portion of your energy expenditure—approximately 20 percent—comes from physical activity. Different people use more or less, depending on how active their lifestyle is. Then about 10 percent is used toward thermogenesis, which has to do with the digestive process. I mention thermogenesis because the body actually uses calories to digest the food you eat.

HOW MUCH FUEL DO YOU NEED?

So how much fuel does your body require? It's not as easy to figure out as with a car. With your car, you know it's full when you hear and feel the "click" that turns off the gas pump. If there were no shutoff "click," the gas would just spill out all over the ground. Research has shown that when you're young, the mind does "click" and tell you, "That's enough. Stop eating." But some children never develop this click, and unfortunately, through different circumstances in life, some of us learn to override that mental click and simply overeat all the time as adults. And so for some of us, we can't rely on our mind to click and tell us we're full. That's the way it was with me. When I was a child I often did not know when I was going to have my next meal, so I would eat as much as possible at every opportunity. In essence, I overrode my body's signal to stop eating in order to survive.

If our bodies won't automatically tell us when we're full, we need to learn to manually regulate our food intake another way so that we can lose the weight we're shooting for right now. We need to pay attention to how much fuel the body requires, just like you would have to know how many gallons it takes to fill up a car if the fuel meter was broken. I had to figure out how many calories it takes to fill up my body for the day's journey. If I don't know this number, when I start to overfuel my body, the fuel just pours over to my sides and my hips and waist, just as if I were overfilling my car with gasoline.

THE MOST IMPORTANT NUMBER IN WEIGHT LOSS

I think you can begin to see that the most important number here is not bench press reps or heart rate or fat grams. The number we need to know in order to be successful in weight loss has to do with our bodies' fuel requirements. The fuel requirement for your body is calculated as your resting metabolic rate, or RMR. In a nutshell, it's the number of calories that your body burns a day while at total rest.

The most important thing to understand if we want to Lose It Fast and Lose It Forever is this concept of RMR. To make it easier to remember, I call it my Personal Daily Fuel Goal. Once I'd figured out this number, all the other elements of weight loss fell into place. I'm not being overdramatic when I say that understanding my Personal Daily Fuel Goal and how it affects weight loss and maintenance has made me the weight loss success I am today. Living by this number has regulated what I eat and how much I exercise, and guarded me against the dreaded lose-gain-lose-gain cycle.

The Personal Daily Fuel Goal varies from person to person because we are all shaped differently. Someone who is four feet tall requires less energy than someone who is six feet tall. A female requires less energy than a male. An older person requires less energy than a younger person, because older people tend to lose muscle mass and muscles consume more energy than fat. Occupation makes a difference, too, as a bank teller will likely burn fewer calories on the job than a construction worker. An athlete will burn more calories while playing her sport than a couch potato will burn while watching her on TV.

It is critical that we know our Personal Daily Fuel Goal. If you consume more calories than your body requires on a daily basis, you will gain weight. I can testify to the truth of this scientific fact. Fifteen years after I left college, I was 150 pounds overweight. But like most people, I didn't just wake up and find myself an entire person heavier than I should have been. No, it took many years of increased basketball watching and decreased basketball playing. More extra helpings and less exercise.

It took many years of Friday-night cheese fries. But before I answer the questions I asked at the beginning of the chapter, I need to explain how a little butter, a little cheese, a little bread, and a little ignorance can put you into the "airplane lap belt extender" category.

You may have heard this before:

3500 calories equals 1 pound.

Remember, a calorie is a unit of energy. You may be saying to yourself, "I would never overeat by 3500 calories! No way!" Let me put it a different way. Overeating your Daily Fuel Goal by just 100 calories a day means you will overeat by 36,500 calories per year. Can you still do division like a fifth grader? Never mind, I'll do it for you:

An extra 36,500 calories equals 10 pounds of weight gained a year.

Let me repeat that because there is a lot of confusion out there: If we overeat by simply 100 calories a day, we're going to gain 10 pounds a year. That 100 calories a day breaks down to:

- One tablespoon of regular mayo on a sandwich
- One pat of butter on your pancakes
- One can of soda
- The top half of a hamburger bun

Think about that. If we overeat our Daily Fuel Goal by one tablespoon of regular mayo a day, we could gain ten pounds a year. And that's how we get fat without knowing how it happens.

OVERFUELING

Remember my typical Friday night meal at the beginning of this chapter? That is a great way to demonstrate this process of slow weight gain. I thank God for my time on *The Biggest Loser,* because this amazing discovery helped save my life.

When I arrived at the ranch, I was given a life-changing book, a calorie counter. As I began to flip through that book, the first thing I did was to investigate my typical Friday night.

When I looked up just these two items—the cheese fries and the hot-buttered movie popcorn with extra butter—in the calorie counter I was shocked at what I had been doing to myself. How many calories do you think are in those two food items alone?

It turns out that the large, hot-buttered movie popcorn by itself was 1500 calories. And there are 2900 calories in that one serving of cheese fries. If you are like I was, these are just numbers. The key is to put those numbers in context. So let's do that.

The Old Pete—or Big Sexy as I like to call him—was over 416

pounds. For me to maintain that weight at 416 pounds, I needed to eat approximately 3500 calories a day. That's right, 3500 calories each and every day to maintain that sexy, svelte figure.

So how many calories did I have for my typical Friday night feast? If you add just those two items together, that's 4400 calories. How many did I need for the day? 3500. So the Old Pete went over what my body required by over 900 calories through just these two foods alone.

Here's the question I want you to ask yourself: Did I lose weight or gain weight that day? If you've done the math, you understand that I gained weight that day. And I haven't even told you what I had for breakfast, lunch, and dinner.

The reason so many of us struggle with our weight is because we have no understanding of how much fuel our body requires on a daily basis. We've heard of things like "calories in, calories out" or that "you need to look at the calorie label on your food." Both of those statements are true, but most people do not understand calories *in context*, so the knowledge does not help them. The context is that you only need so many calories a day to fuel your body. If you go over that number, you're going to gain weight. If you go under that number, you're going to lose weight.

There's one caveat here: Carbohydrates have to be treated specially. I will explain more about that in future chapters. Right now, I just need you to understand the basic concept of a Personal Daily Fuel Goal. Hopefully you understand why I was gaining weight each and every time I went out on Friday night before I understood this concept. Now you need to take that information and figure it out for yourself. You have to figure out your Personal Daily Fuel Goal so you can pursue losing it fast and losing it forever.

CALCULATING YOUR RMR

So how do you figure out your Personal Daily Fuel Goal? You have a couple of different options. I'm going to give you several, including my personal recommendation.

The most accurate—and most expensive—way is to go to a professional lab and have your RMR tested. You can undergo formal testing at many labs, hospitals, and health clubs around the country. I did this. It was great. They put a mask over my face as I lay on my back in a dark, quiet room. They turned the lights off and just let me rest as I listened to New Age whale sounds. I felt like I was communicating with my family members. As I rested, the equipment was calculating how many calories my body was burning by measuring the amount of oxygen I was using.

The good news is that there is an easier way for you to do it. All you have to do is go to www.PeteThomas.com to help you to calculate your current and goal weight RMR. I didn't want to stay at my current weight, so I had a current and a goal weight RMR. Go and figure out your RMR right now. Then I want you to memorize your goal weight RMR as your Personal Daily Fuel Goal.

There are a few different ways to calculate RMRs, but in my opinion the most accurate formula for calculating your Personal Daily Fuel Goal is the Mifflin RMR formula. You can find the actual equation online at many websites, including mine, so I won't go over it here.

If you can't get to a computer, there are a couple of other ways to calculate your Personal Daily Fuel Goal. First, there's the quick and dirty "simple" formula. This is the least reliable method, but it will give you an approximate number to work with. All you have to do is multiply your current body weight by ten and then add your current body weight back in. For example, a 150-pound person would take that and multiply by ten—that's 1500, plus 150 equals 1,650 calories a day. This isn't very accurate, but it will give you a place to start until you can get a more precise number.

SUPER-SECRET RANCH INSIDER INFO

Read this slowly: When I was on *The Biggest Loser,* I took in between 1600 and 1800 calories a day because I was in *Biggest Loser* weight loss mode. When I got home, I took in between 1800 and 2000 calories a day because I was still trying to drop some pounds, but not as quickly as on the show. The month before I went back to the finale, I took in 2500 calories a day because, even though I wanted to lose those last few pounds, I was working out so incredibly hard that I needed the extra fuel to keep my energy up.

Now I take in approximately 2400 to 2500 calories a day as I maintain my goal weight; this includes a good, hard workout six days a week.

I learned that there are some amazing things that go along with this calorie concept. As I was going along my weight loss journey, I learned how to eat fewer calories a day without giving up the amount of food I wanted to eat. This is amazing! As I began to work out even harder, I was able to increase my calories. And now that I've hit my goal weight, I'm able to elevate my calories even further because I'm maintaining my weight.

FACTORING IN ACTIVITY

I hope you've already made a printout of your RMR (resting metabolic rate) from my website, because I want to talk to you a little bit about that. On your printout, there are a couple of different things. One is your goal weight RMR. After that, you see your current and your goal weight AMR, or active metabolic rate. That is where we factor in your activity level. The active metabolic rate is the additional number of calories your body burns based upon your occupation and exercise level. For instance, as I mentioned earlier, if you have an active job like being a postal carrier, you require more calories than someone who sits at a desk all day. A "weekend warrior" who plays basketball on Saturdays is going to need fewer calories than a professional athlete.

Be careful not to overestimate the number of calories that your occupation requires you to burn. The reason is, as you begin any job, the body has to adjust. So as you begin a job, you may burn extra calories. But over time your body begins to adapt and you will burn fewer and fewer calories on a daily basis from doing the same activity. If you want to be safe like me, just use your RMR, or Personal Daily Fuel Goal, and ignore the activity factor completely!

Learning your Personal Daily Fuel Goal can truly change your life, as it did mine. But I'm sure some of you are thinking, "Oh, great, another number. Now what do I do with this?" That's a great question. The key to success is not just storing up information in the brain but applying it to real-life situations. I was able to build my life around this knowledge, and it has allowed me to Lose It Forever. But to really use the knowledge, it has to work in every situation in life. And it really does work. I am about to show you how this Personal Daily Fuel Goal can work for you in every situation in your life as well.

EATING FOR LIFE

It's the perfect time to share with you my number one principle of nutrition. Notice I said nutrition, not diet, because I prefer that you pursue something that you can do forever.

My number one principle of nutrition is: Never, ever, EVER start a diet that you can't maintain for the rest of your life.

What I want you to do is move from dieting to eating for life. Many of us—myself included—have struggled with weight loss for a long time; we've struggled with eating poorly over the years, and so we just can't be on a diet. We have to be on a way of life. There is a big difference between pursuing a diet and pursuing a lifestyle. One is doomed to failure; the other is destined for success.

Lose It Fast, Lose It Forever is about creating a new you. It is about creating a new reality by challenging you to make some modifications to the way you eat in the coming chapters. Don't worry, this isn't one of those fad diets where you will get half of your daily caloric needs by eating only dried squid or something like that. I'm not going to dictate the amount or type of food at all, to be honest, but you will need to make some changes to Lose It Forever.

MANAGE YOUR MOUTH

If you're going to maintain your weight loss long-term—and by that I mean the rest of your life—then you are going to have to learn how to Manage Your Mouth. I'm not talking about changing the way you talk (although that is important, and we covered that in Step 1), I mean that you have to get control over what kind of food goes into your mouth.

In a general sense, there are only two types of diet programs. Well, three, if you count mine, which is a hybrid of the two. But in general, most plans fall under one of two different categories: counting plans and set plans.

Counting plans are where you're counting calories, or you're counting carbohydrates, or maybe you're counting points or grams of sodium. The point is, you're counting something every time you eat. This kind of plan has pros and cons, which I will explain in a minute.

The other type of plan is a set plan. A set plan is where you're prescribed a certain thing for breakfast, a certain thing for lunch, and a certain thing for dinner, as well as certain snacks. Again, there are some very popular set plans that you've probably seen on TV or in magazines, or even tried yourself.

The truth is, all diets can work temporarily. Even a starvation diet will help you lose weight if you stick to it. The question really is, will these diets work for you long-term? To help you figure that out, let's go in depth into a couple of these different programs.

WHERE THE FLUBBER MEETS THE ROAD

Atkins, the South Beach Diet, and Weight Watchers are examples of counting plans. A counting plan, again, is where you have to count calories, or carbohydrates, or something else. These are good for restricting the number of calories or carbs that go into your mouth, so they have some value.

I have several problems with counting plans. The first is that they can dumb you down. These plans may not actually teach you much about nutrition. It's fine to understand the point value of a product, but it's better to understand the nutritional component of the product. For instance, if you are counting points through a system like Weight Watchers, a single point can range from between 80 and 120 calories. Progresso Light Soup is zero points, although it does have calories. I have asked myself, "What is the calculation that ultimately determines these points? Are these points based on any nutritional values?" Calories are simple and fundamental. I cannot only understand them as units of energy, but I can build on this knowledge to create a lifestyle.

I've had students who have done counting in other plans. And in those programs, you're rewarded for any extra exercise that you put in. That's good, but they reward you by allowing you more food than you're otherwise allowed to eat. This can at times sabotage your weight loss efforts, as it did for my students.

The other problem with counting plans is a logistical one. What, for instance, are you going to do with your counting plan when you go to Chicago, like I've done, and you sit down and have a slice of Giordano's

Chicago-style, deep-dish pizza? When you have that pizza, you have no idea how many points or how many carbs are in that slice of pizza. What is the value of your counting plan in that real world situation?

Now let's talk about set plans, like Jenny Craig or Nutrisystem. These plans tell you what to eat for breakfast, what to eat for lunch, and what to eat for dinner. Because they are very specific and they work well for a certain amount of time, they are very popular plans.

But the plans I just mentioned do not teach you how to eat, they only tell you what to eat. And what are you going to do when the food that you're supposed to eat is not available? Let's say that you go on a vacation to Las Vegas and the Grand Canyon. You're enjoying your day out in nature. You're hiking around, burning calories, and about lunchtime you start to get hungry. Really hungry.

What are you going to do when your special food that's supposed to be refrigerated is not available in the Grand Canyon? You eat what's available, like everyone else. Well, I have news for you: If you don't eat the food on the plan, you're not on the plan. So set plans have obvious limitations.

THE COOKIE DIET . . . NO THANKS

Most diets are not sustainable for a lifetime. That's because they operate on the basis of restriction alone. Let me explain. You may have heard of the Master Cleanse (also called the Lemonade Diet because it's made of maple syrup, cayenne pepper, and lemon juice) or one of several "cookie" diets.

The Master Cleanse is famous among Hollywood stars because it helps people shed pounds quickly. On the cookie diet, which has understandable appeal, you have a cookie for breakfast, a cookie for lunch, and a regular meal for dinner. It's very popular in certain parts of the country. And like I said, these plans work for some people.

But here is the key. They only work in one way—restriction. You're going to lose weight from caloric or carbohydrate restriction. If you're not making any real changes to your life, you're just temporarily restricting these things from your body. If the diet is not sustainable for you in your life, then it's just not a good diet. You have to be able to stick with the diet in any and all circumstances for it to be long-term. The bottom line is that you need to have a plan that's going to work in your real life for your entire life.

HOW TO LOSE WEIGHT FAST AND FOREVER

The only way to lose 1 pound is by eating less than your Personal Daily Fuel Goal daily and weekly. For one week, I'm going to ask you to reduce your daily caloric intake by 500 calories—every day for seven days. That's going to equal 3500 calories, or 1 pound of weight loss this week. There is nothing magical about this number, but it is the most common recommendation—reduce your caloric intake just enough to shed 1 pound a week.

If you want to achieve quicker weight loss—if you want to Lose It Fast—it's quite simple. You can do what I did; I *lowered* my Personal Daily Fuel Goal to achieve a greater caloric deficit. I didn't just stick with 500 fewer calories a day for a pound a week. No, as I explained above, I lowered my Fuel Goal to 1600 to 1800 calories a day for *Biggest Loser*–type results. The reason I lowered my Personal Daily Fuel Goal so drastically is because I had so much extra weight to lose and could do so safely. So I was able to lower my Daily Fuel Goal to accelerate the weight loss. Once I had lost the weight, I adjusted it to a more normal level.

As a caution, I want you to understand that you should not cut your Personal Daily Fuel Goal too low. Common recommendations state that men should not go below 1600 calories a day and women should not reduce their calories below 1200 calories a day. That's one reason I don't like those weird diets I mentioned earlier, which often take you down to 800 calories a day. You don't want your body to think you're starving it, because it will fight back by producing certain hormones that will lead to extra weight regain. We will talk more about hormones in Chapter 7.

SECRET WEAPON

If you follow the guidelines in this program, you will lose weight. What I'm about to explain to you will accelerate the timing of that weight loss. It's one of my "secret weapons" in the fight against flab.

I call this secret weapon caloric cycling, and it's an advanced concept. To explain it, I will use exercise as an analogy. When it comes to working out, you've got to change your workouts to keep your body guessing. The concept is that you don't want to do the same exercises over and over because your muscles will adapt. This is not really a new concept. When the muscles adapt, you stop seeing improvements in a particular muscle. The body becomes accustomed to what you're doing and it says, "Thank you. We'll stick with this. This doesn't stress me out at all." But when it comes to exercise, stressing the body is actually good for you. So you need to change your exercise routine to see growth.

When it comes to eating, the body is just as efficient. If you give it the same thing each and every day, your body will become accustomed to it. For instance, if you give it the same number of calories and the same type of food every day, the body becomes super-efficient at burning it. It's similar to exercise: Walk around the block every day, and the first couple of days you're going to use a lot of energy; then it's going to get easier as the body adapts.

In the same way, the more you eat foods with exactly the same number of calories, the more your body will become accustomed to it and learn to burn this amount more efficiently. The result is that you'll use less energy consuming and digesting it. That's why we want to vary the amount of calories we take in on a daily basis. Below you can see two examples of this particular method of caloric cycling.

Monday	Tuesday	Wednesday	Thursday	Friday	Saturday	Sunday
Caloric Cycling Example Based on 1800/Day (used for weight loss)						
1620	1980	1530	1980	1620	1800	2070
- 10% RMRx.90	+ 10% RMRx1.10	- 15% RMRx.85	+ 10% RMRx1.10	- 10% RMRx.90	+ 0% RMR	+ 15% RMRx1.15
Caloric Cycling Example Based on 2500/Day (used for maintenance) Increase your calories cleanly, stay within your calories, watch the carbs (sugar), and enjoy life!						
2250	2750	2125	2750	2250	2500	2875

THE FIRST EXAMPLE is based on a RMR of 1800 calories. On Monday, I would start with my RMR, but take in 10 percent fewer calories than my RMR. On Tuesday, I would take in 10 percent more calories. On

Wednesday, I would take in 15 percent fewer calories. On Thursday, I would take in 10 percent more. On Friday, 10 percent less. On Saturday, I would hit my RMR exactly right. And then on Sunday, I would take in 15 percent more.

Following this regimen will accomplish a couple things in your diet journey. One, you have a little bit more food on the weekends, which may help you emotionally. Two, I believe that you keep the body guessing because it doesn't know exactly how many calories are coming.

In maintenance mode, I'm consuming approximately 2500 calories a day, which is about my RMR now. So on Monday, I'll take in 2250 calories; on Tuesday, 2750 calories; on Wednesday, 2125 calories; on Thursday, 2750 calories; on Friday, 2250 calories; on Saturday, 2500 calories; and on Sunday, 2875 calories.

You will get amazing results if you try this. But again, it's an advanced concept that is easier to grasp once you've practiced modifying your daily calories. In Step 3: Your Pursuit, we will incorporate this concept to accelerate our weight loss when we're trying to reach a particular goal.

THE DANGER OF UNDEREATING

Overeating is a huge problem, as you know. But I often deal with people who are undereating—mostly women. They follow a similar pattern, taking in only 800 or 900 calories a day, which would make you think they are losing weight. But they aren't losing; they are gaining.

First of all, they don't eat any breakfast or lunch. Then they turn around and eat a large dinner with 800 or 900 calories, and that's it for the day. They can't understand why they keep gaining weight or why they can't lose weight.

As I learned on the ranch, the human body is amazing. It will not allow you to lose weight when you do things poorly. The body can go into a catabolic state, where it thinks it's in starvation mode, and will actually consume bones and muscle for energy while holding on to fat. Starvation mode is when you undereat the number of calories that your body requires a day. When you undereat, when you go below those 1200- or 1600-calorie limits, your body releases a hormone called cortisol that can actually inhibit weight loss. So we do not want to go below 1200 or 1600 calories a day, depending on your gender, because we don't want this hormone to be released.

While we do want to create a caloric deficit weekly, you should never go below the thresholds I mentioned for any extended period of time. Extended means more than a couple of days. I mean, sometimes you have a day where you're simply busy and you didn't eat all your food; that's understandable. And some people fast for religious reasons; that's fine for a short period of time.

But when you undereat, you'll have to be careful of the rebound effect, which we'll talk more about more in Chapter 9. Suffice it to say that there is a rebound effect that happens when you begin to undereat for any period of time and then you go back to normal eating. Your body thought you were starving and wants to make sure it has enough extra fuel to survive another starvation period. So be aware of that.

YOU CAN DO THIS

I hope you're beginning to think about some of the changes that need to occur for you to begin to lose weight. I know it seems a little daunting right now, but don't worry. In the next chapters, I'm going to introduce a revolutionary idea that was very exciting to me. It will help you to apply the information you have learned so far to truly Lose It Forever.

KEY POINTS

1. Pete's Weight Loss 101:
   - Lose weight = reduce calories
   - Reduce calories = reduce fats, carbs, and proteins (macronutrients)
   - Lose weight further = reduce calories and carb ratio
2. The most important thing to understand if you want to lose weight quickly and permanently is your Personal Daily Fuel Goal.
3. Number one principle of nutrition is: Never, ever, EVER start a diet you can't maintain for the rest of your life.

CHAPTER 5 CHALLENGES

New Challenges | Print Out Your Personal Daily Fuel Goal from My Website and Memorize It

You should have already made a printout of your present weight and your goal weight Personal Daily Fuel Goal. If you haven't, do it now. You can get it from PeteThomas.com. Make sure you memorize it.

Begin to Make Small Modifications

I told you in this chapter that one extra pat of butter on your pancakes can be the 100 calories that make you go over your Daily Fuel Goal for the day. Start thinking about some small changes you can make to eliminate a few calories here and there. It might be as easy as drinking diet soda or having a glass of water instead of soda. Write down three small changes you could make to create a calorie deficit.

Ongoing Challenges | Get a Calorie Counter

You should have already purchased a good calorie counter or be using an online or smart phone alternative. If you don't have one, you'll need one. It will become your best friend as you discover what's really in the food you and your family consume!

Continue Journaling

Creating an open mind-set will be easier as you share how you're feeling in your LIF2 Success Journal. So continue to write about your connection with food and how well you are Mastering Your Mind.

In addition, now that we have learned about calories and Personal Daily Fuel Goal, this information will help us figure out how many calories we are presently consuming. We'll be able to figure out—are we LOSING weight daily or GAINING weight daily? You've already been recording everything that goes into your mouth; now it's time to research how many calories are in what we're eating and record it. The only way to know what you need to change is to record how many calories you're consuming. So write it out in your journal every day.

Communicate with Your Team

We're moving into a new stage of weight loss now, stepping it up a notch, so we need to be sure to let our team know how we're doing and how they can help us.

Review Your Lists

In Step 1: Your Power, you created your Personal Success Statement. Also, you were asked to memorize your top 3 reasons for losing weight (your Personal Power Goals) from your Top 10 List. Now you need to review your Personal Success Statement and your "top 3" from your Top 10 daily so that you can remember why you want to lose weight in the first place. Keeping these things in the "front of your mind" will help you to create a willing mind-set.

Weigh Weekly and Measure Monthly

Remember to keep weighing in weekly and measuring monthly to check your progress. If you do it at the same time every week, it will become part of your routine—one of those Forever Habits we were talking about.

"My initial goal weight was 185 pounds, but I've passed that and now I'm about 175 pounds. So I've lost about 70 pounds. It's absolutely a life change. And I plan on doing it forever, because I still eat the things I like. I've learned to modify what I like rather than deprive myself of the things I want."

—STEVE, LIF2 STUDENT

CHAPTER

MODIFICATION NOT STARVATION

TO DEMONSTRATE MY POINT THAT LOSE IT FAST, LOSE IT FOREVER IS a combination of the two types of diet plans I explained in Chapter 5, I need to tell you a little story.

On a spring day several years ago, I went to Detroit to get my hair cut at my barbershop. My barber and I were discussing different things, as folks do in a barbershop. I mentioned that I had seen this incredible movie a few days ago. "It is violent," I said, "but it is a great, great movie. She said, "Yeah, I saw that movie last night with the kids."

My first thought was, "Wow! This is a really violent movie for kids." I asked her what theater had allowed her to watch the movie with her kids, since it was rated R. She said, "No, I watched the movie at home.

We can't afford to go to the theater anymore, so I bought the DVD." I thought that was odd, considering that the movie had only been released in theaters two days before. So I asked her how she watched the movie at home and she said, "I bought a bootleg copy at the liquor-drugstore."

I had never heard of that kind of a store, so I asked her where it was. She told me it was around the corner, and sure enough, when I was done, I went around the corner and found the store. It was an old drugstore from the early 1900s that had been converted into a liquor store. And sure enough, they were selling bootleg copies of the movie we had discussed during the haircut. I understand that it is hypocritical, not to mention illegal, for a person who claims to be a Christian to buy a bootleg movie, but sometimes people in desperate financial situations do things they wouldn't normally do. Especially when the movie I bought that day was *The Passion of the Christ*. Ouch!

BEHAVIOR MODIFICATION

I tell you this story not to get myself in trouble but to illustrate a point about how people will change their behavior when times get hard. Say you like to go to the movies, but the economy forces you to tighten your belt and stop going to the theater every Friday night. What would you do?

You would modify your behavior. You probably wouldn't give up watching movies; you would just watch them in a different way. You would either go to the matinee, or you would rent a DVD, or you would go to the dollar movie. Hopefully you would not go to the liquor-drugstore in Detroit and buy them bootleg! But in short, you would modify your behavior to fit within your budget.

YOUR CALORIE BUDGET

I want you to start thinking of calories as a sort of edible money. We have an account full of calories that we can spend every day—which is the number we talked about in Chapter 5, our Personal Daily Fuel Goal. We have a daily and a weekly budget of calories, so we can simply modify our eating behavior to fit our food into our caloric budget. I call this concept Modification Not Starvation.

If you follow my principles, you won't feel like I did when I tried those other diet programs—hungry all the time. I never felt like I ate enough food. I am a big guy and I need a lot of food to feel full. The good news: My program is not going to restrict the amount of food you eat; you're just going to modify it so that you eat within your caloric goals.

In the Homework Challenge at the end of this section, we're going to create an actual caloric checkbook. It's an exercise that will help you Manage Your Mouth, because you'll know just how many calories you've consumed so far today, as well as how many you have yet to eat in your caloric bank account. The nice thing about this bank account is that we can spend it every day and it renews magically so that we can spend it again tomorrow!

Unlike many short-term diet programs, this one is not going to restrict or forbid all of the foods that you like. That's why my program will help you for the rest of your life. You will modify your favorite foods so that you can have all you want and still Lose It Forever. Life got incredibly fun for me when I hit upon this and started playing with different foods. I found out that I could still eat just about everything that I wanted to eat and I would not have to go hungry.

SECRET REVEALED—BIGGEST LOSER FOODS

But before we go any further, I've got to let you in on a little secret. People have always asked me, "What secret foods did you guys eat on the ranch?" They think that we had trained chefs there to prepare special foods that were hidden from the public eye. So I'm going to give you some of the super-duper-secret foods we ate at the ranch. This is from my personal food inventory that I took with me from *The Biggest Loser* Ranch. Are you ready? Here is what I ate:

milk, yogurt, cheese, sour cream, Reddi-wip, ricotta cheese, chicken, beef, salmon fillets, tuna steaks, turkey burgers, shrimp, ham, bacon, fish, breakfast sausages, apples, pears, raspberries, strawberries, plums, peaches, cucumbers, green/red/yellow bell peppers, broccoli, cauliflower, cereal, oats, tortillas, rice, pinto beans, black beans, lima beans, peanut butter, almonds, walnuts, cashews, pistachios, peanuts, bread, oil, butter, pepper, olive oil, ketchup, barbecue sauce, tomato sauce, mustard, jam, salad dressing, Jell-O, hot chocolate, popcorn, Fudgsicles, Popsicles, Creamsicles, eggs, soda pop

That sounds like a whole bunch of regular food, doesn't it? You're right, it is. However, there was one difference: The key was the caloric content of the foods we ate. We ate a lot of fruits, vegetables, and lean protein, and the low-fat or sugar-free or lean version of all of the other foods. So we ate all familiar foods, but they were leaner quality or better portioned. We never went hungry at the ranch, nor did we eat anything special or odd.

That was important, because when we undereat, it leads to an increase in bad hormones, and it can also lead to bingeing. Our goal is to Lose It Forever, not follow one diet after another.

One day Jillian was working us out in the gym when this very strange conversation took place:

> Jillian: Guys, your workout sucks today. How have you been eating?
>
> Guys: We didn't eat much. We had to film stuff for production today.
>
> Jillian: G&% #@#$##. Flim Flarn Filth Flarn Production! Workout is canceled! Get out of here and go eat!
>
> Guys: But then you won't be able to give us our workout!
>
> Jillian: I don't care, go eat!

Yes, Jillian canceled the workout and made us go eat. We contestants became so conscious about getting in enough calories that I remember Matt (the eventual winner of my season) and I actually splitting a pound of hamburger at 11:00 p.m. to make sure we got in all of our calories for the day. And we were upset about it.

Think about that, fat people mad because we had to eat! But I came to understand firsthand that undereating leads to serious problems for people who are trying to lose weight. We talked about this in the last chapter.

PETE'S MODIFICATIONS TO EVERYDAY FOOD

Having said all that, undereating was definitely not my problem. No, I was one of the many overeaters out there. So I had to begin to think of food in a new way.

The basic question is: How do we modify our favorite foods so that we eat until we're full and never go hungry? We do it by making intelligent, caloric-based substitutions. I'm going to show you some of my favorite substitutions. If you love food like I do, this discussion should get you excited about the possibilities.

I'll start with eggs, because people associate eggs with breakfast. You could have two eggs for 140 calories or you could have *four servings* of Egg Beaters for that same 140 calories. That's because one egg is 70 calories, while one serving of Egg Beaters is only 35 calories. So if you like eggs for breakfast, you can have the 140 calories in two eggs, or you can modify your breakfast and have four servings of Egg Beaters for that same 140 calories. Or if you just have to have the real egg taste, combine a real egg with two serving of Egg Beaters. See how that works?

Next, let's look at bacon. Two slices of regular bacon are about 80 calories each, or 160 calories total. You could modify that by eating *eight slices* of turkey bacon for that same 160 calories. Could you get used to the slightly different taste in order to lose weight and keep your favorite breakfast food? That's a no-brainer for me.

As another example, you could have one regular 4-ounce burger for 300 calories or you could have *two* 96 percent lean hamburgers of the same size for the same 300 calories.

It is amazing what we can do to fill ourselves up with our favorite foods and cut calories at the same time:

- We could have one liter of regular soda for around 250 calories or we could have an infinite number of liters of diet soda for exactly zero calories. Eventually I'd like to transition you to mostly water, but let's not get crazy while you're still at the beginning of the process!

- We could have one pat of butter for 90 calories or we could have one spray of butter substitute like I Can't Believe It's Not Butter! for 1 calorie.
- We could have one large, hot-buttered movie popcorn for 1500 calories or we could have the same amount of hot air-popped popcorn for less than 200 calories with a good-tasting butter substitute.
- We could have ⅓ cup of syrup for 300 calories, or we could have ⅓ cup of light syrup for 150 calories.
- We could have one tablespoon of mayo for 100 calories or we could replace that with one tablespoon of light mayo for just 50 calories.

Try to put these suggestions into context. Remember that if you overeat your Personal Daily Fuel Goal by 100 calories a day, you are going to consume an additional 36,500 calories a year and you're guaranteed to put on 10 pounds a year.

The goal with Modification Not Starvation is to find the right balance between calories and taste. For example, instead of having regular jam, try low-sugar jam, and from there try sugar-free or unsweetened jam. If you can go all the way down to no sugar, you're going to save yourself calories for some other food. The many good sugar substitutes on the market right now are going to make this much easier. I use the artificial sweetener Splenda because I like the taste and it contains no calories. However, many nutritionally savvy people, including my mentor Jillian, prefer sweeteners that are produced from natural sources, like xylitol and stevia. You can experiment and determine which is best for you.

A BREAKFAST EXAMPLE

Before I was cast on *The Biggest Loser,* this is what I used to eat for breakfast:

9 slices of bacon × 80 calories each = 720 calories
4 eggs × 70 calories = 280 calories
16 ounces grapefruit juice = 180 calories
Total Old Pete breakfast = 1180 calories

So how has that changed? Now I eat:

9 slices of turkey bacon × 20 calories each = 180 calories
4 servings of Egg Beaters × 35 calories = 140 calories
16 ounces Crystal Light Ruby Red = 10 calories
Total New Pete breakfast = 330 calories

My breakfast alone has gone from 1180 calories all the way down to 330! So I saved somewhere around 850 calories—and I'm eating just as much—simply by using this principle of Modification Not Starvation. Could you form a Forever Habit and Lose It Forever with this kind of modification? You bet. This is an amazing principle, and if you understand it, you're going to be slim for the rest of your life.

You must experiment to see what foods you like, then modify, modify, modify. Chances are, you will not love everything you eat at first, but you can modify or substitute your foods and save a lot of calories in your budget. Food companies are getting better at producing tasty, low-calorie alternatives as more people look for them. Over time you will get better at selecting these alternatives to the foods you normally eat.

In the Challenges section at the end of this chapter, I am going to ask you to make some simple modifications to the foods you normally eat, keeping in mind the principle of Modification Not Starvation. Make some adjustments and try to find that balance between taste and calories I talked about.

MODIFYING FOR LIFE

I told you that my weight loss plan is more of a lifestyle change than a diet plan. Modifying our foods does not end when we reach our long-term goal weight. We're not going back to the way we used to eat—we're moving on to healthier food habits.

At first, we modify only to form that Forever Habit and lose that next pound. Truthfully, we are only "eating for weight loss." After we see success in that area, we start modifying because we're "eating for health," or you might call it "eating for life," which will involve many more natural, whole, and unprocessed foods. So we are really modifying in two steps. I'll give you an example.

We all know that we should be drinking water. Soda pop is bad for you, and you should be drinking a lot more water. But we've become so used to eating everything with flavor that many of us can't go cold turkey and just start drinking water. It's okay to move from regular pop to diet pop, and then from diet pop to flavored water, and from there to regular water. Progress slowly to wean yourself off the harmful stuff until your body adjusts.

You can take your time with this progression. Small steps and small changes. Around southeast Michigan we have lots of automotive plants. The car companies talk about the principle of *kaizen*, where you make little changes that add up to a big difference. As of this writing, I am seven years off *The Biggest Loser,* but it was just a few years ago that I started to make the transition to eating for health rather than just eating for weight loss. So I've gone from regular soda pop to diet soda pop, and now I drink less and less diet pop and more and more water.

Sugar substitutes, such as those in Crystal Light and diet sodas, play an important role in low-calorie foods, so it's important to have an understanding of these substances. I personally believe that we should use sugar substitutes for the reason they were intended for, to save calories. Over time, however, we should wean ourselves off those, too. For some people, sugar substitutes may increase their cravings for the sweet stuff and make us more susceptible to derailing our new, healthy eating habits. For others, like me, they actually satisfy our cravings while keeping the overall calories lower.

ANOTHER POISON

Understanding the effects of high-fructose corn syrup on the body is another important aspect of eating for health. I remember reading a study concerning college athletes. These athletes worked out between three and four hours a day. They were given jelly beans composed of normal, regular sugars. During the course of the week, those jelly beans were burned up like any other fuel—the body didn't even blink at those calories that came from sugar.

Then the athletes were given the same amount of jelly beans made with high-fructose corn syrup and an amazing thing happened. The athletes began to gain body fat. Why was that? The study concluded that the athletes' bodies did not know how to handle this artificial sugar. High-fructose corn syrup would bypass the normal digestive processes and get passed over into the fat stores. The lesson for us is, whenever possible, avoid high-fructose corn syrup. I can't stress this enough—read your food labels and pay attention to what's in your food!

The whole matter boils down to this: The closer your food is to how God made it, the better. The food industry responded to the government's call to lower fat intake by making such ingredients as high-fructose corn syrup (HFCS). The result, I believe, is that people are worse off with HFCS in their diet than they were with fat. So the important thing is to get as close to the way God made the food as possible. This means vegetables, unprocessed meat and dairy, fruits, and certain grains.

AVOID THE CYCLE OF DEATH

A lot of programs out there are promising quick, miracle cures—either magic surgery or magic foods. I hope you can see by now that there are no magic pills or magic foods. Lose It Fast, Lose It Forever is based on eating real foods with a cap on calories, using the principle of Modification Not Starvation.

This process, which will get easier and easier, will lead to our Losing It Forever as we form Forever Habits that create a 3500-calorie deficit over time. Every day we can spend the calories in our caloric checkbook (which equals your Personal Daily Fuel Goal) by modifying and eating as much as we want within our budget. Our focus should be on calories while keeping a cautious eye on carbohydrates. More about this in Chapter 7.

But through this whole learning process, we need to give ourselves room to fall down and get back up again. Avoid what I call the "cycle of death." That's when we have a bad lunch and we feel so bad about messing up that we end up having a bad dinner. That bad dinner means that we've blown it again, so why not have late-night ice cream? Now that bad lunch has turned into a bad day altogether. And that bad day can easily turn into a bad weekend, which ends up turning into a bad week.

That caloric bank account I talked about should convince you that one bad lunch does not equal a bad dinner, a bad dinner does not equal a bad day, and a bad day does not equal a bad weekend. If you had a flat tire, would you go around and puncture all the other tires on your car? Of course not. You spent too many calories on lunch—okay, adjust your next meal to make up for it and go on to lose that Forever Few so that they never return.

KEY POINTS

- Modification Not Starvation means we can simply modify our eating behavior to fit our food into our caloric budget.
- How do we modify our favorite foods so that we eat until we're full and never go hungry? We do it by making intelligent, caloric-based substitutions.
- One bad lunch does not equal a bad dinner, a bad dinner does not equal a bad day, and a bad day does not equal a bad weekend.

CHAPTER 6 CHALLENGES

Create a Caloric Checkbook

On an index card or piece of paper, or in a computer spreadsheet, make a graph with three columns like this:

What I Ate Today	Number of Calories	Calories Left for Today
		1570 (goal weight RMR)
Whopper with cheese	770	1570 − 770 = 800 left

TAKE THE GOAL weight Personal Daily Fuel Goal you calculated from Chapter 5 and put it in the right-hand column just like you would write your checking account total in a bank checkbook. In the left-hand column below that, write down what you ate for breakfast, lunch, snacks, and dinner, along with the number of calories in these dishes (you can find that in your calorie counter). You won't have to do this forever, but this exercise will get you to think in terms of a "caloric budget." A sample is available at www.PeteThomas.com.

Search Out Modifications to "Major Food Items"

Start searching out lower-calorie, good-tasting alternatives to the foods that you eat. For instance, begin eating lean hamburger rather than regular hamburger. Eat light ice cream rather than the high-fat kind. Write down modifications to ten of your daily foods in your food journal. Put down the item name and calories and then write down the modified item and calories, along with the caloric savings. A simple example would be:

Old Food and Calories	Modified Food and Calories	Calories Saved
Bacon slice—80 calories	Turkey bacon slice—20 calories	60 calories

Trumpet Your Forever Habit or Forever Few Success

As you form a Forever Habit or lose that Forever Few, celebrate by commenting at www.PeteThomas.com. Read the posts of others who've achieved their goal and share your own success.

Start Cleaning Out Your Cupboards

As we modify our daily foods, we need to make sure that we replace our old bad foods with our new finds. Keep in mind we're not starving ourselves; we're employing the principle of Modification Not Starvation. You can take this as slowly or as quickly as you feel you can handle it. It might be a good idea to call a team member over to help you with this sometimes difficult task.

"I struggle with being a binge eater. For me, sugar is like a gateway drug—it leads to cravings, which lead to bingeing. Binges are a big reason I am significantly overweight, and obviously they make losing weight and keeping it off difficult. I've found that minimizing my intake significantly reduces the chances of a binge. LIF2 helped me shift my main nutrition focus away from fat, which I don't even track anymore, to sugar, enabling me to lose 25 pounds over the past nine weeks."

—JIM, LIF2 STUDENT

CHAPTER

7

CORRECT CALORIES, CAUTIOUS CARBS

FOR SEVERAL YEARS, I WORKED AS A SOFTWARE SUPPORT TECHNICIAN and computer programmer for a nationwide book distributor. My habit at breakfast was to eat two bowls of Frosted Flakes with the milk up to the rim of the bowl. Or I'd "eat healthy" and have Raisin Bran cereal with sugar sprinkled on top. I would eat that at home and then, as I was budgeting my finances, I would bring $5 for lunch.

The problem was that I was spending the $5 in the vending machines by 10:30 a.m. and then borrowing $7 from my friend Richard for a fast-food lunch. Then I would have more snacks in the afternoon and go home and have a typically carb-heavy American meal for dinner. By the time payday rolled around I would have gained a small amount of weight and owed Richard a small portion of my check. I did this over and over for years, and my bank account shrank while my waistline continued to grow.

Why did I continue to do this? Three reasons, really. The first is that I didn't know I was overeating my body's daily calorie needs and thereby gaining a tiny bit of weight each day. The second reason is that I had formed a carbohydrate addiction without realizing it. While there is a pile of evidence that your body and your brain can become addicted to sugar, there are still some researchers who call sugar addiction a "soft" addiction. But sugar in the bloodstream stimulates the "pleasure center" of the brain that releases the hormone serotonin, the "feel good" hormone. Once your body gets used to this temporarily pleasurable feeling, it wants more of the same, especially when blood sugar gets low. Eventually it takes more and more sugar to achieve that "sugar high." I will talk more about this in the coming pages. The third reason I continued to eat this way is that I did not know there was a better, healthier way to eat. The healthy choices I did hear about back then sounded too complicated or too disgusting to adopt for a lifetime.

The bottom line is that I did not know about the principles that we're going to discuss in this chapter: the macronutrients, the truth about carbohydrates, and the Four Cs.

A CARB BY ANY OTHER NAME

As I explained in Chapter 5, your body takes the food you eat, breaks it down, and converts it to energy to fuel all your daily activities. The energy in food is measured in calories. These units of energy come packaged in three different macronutrients: carbohydrates, fats, and proteins.

Macronutrients, which are called "macro" because the body needs a lot of them, provide the nutrients we need for growth, metabolism, and body functions. Micronutrients, which do not contain calories, are the vitamins and minerals we need in very small amounts. For instance, salt is a mineral necessary for our bodies. We need salt to regulate our body's water content and to help with certain processes of our nervous system. It can also enhance the flavor of food. However, studies show that too much salt can cause major problems, like high blood pressure and stroke, so we have to be careful not to put more than we need into our system.

Salt also affects weight loss, which I will address when I talk about the "white poisons" later in this chapter.

Although we all get our nutrition from the three macronutrients, we can choose what ratio of those food types we consume. The choices you make regarding your macronutrient ratio will affect your mood, your weight loss, and your health in general. There is a lot of information—and misinformation—out there about carbohydrates, so I want to address that now. There are entire books written on this subject, so I can't address in depth the many studies that have been done on carbs, but I will provide an overview so that you can make intelligent choices as you move toward preparing your own Perfect Personalized Forever Meal Plan.

IS EASIEST ALWAYS BEST?

For most people, a majority of their food falls into the carbohydrate category. This includes foods that are primarily carbs, like breads, cereals, pasta, rice, cookies, baked goods, French fries, potato chips, fruit drinks, and sugared sodas. Some foods, like ice cream, contain fat and protein but still have a lot of carbs because of their high sugar content. Even fruits and some vegetables are considered carbs. I advocate reducing carbs in almost every situation, but it's important to understand carbs as you develop your Forever Habits.

Carbohydrates—which are basically sugars and starches—are the easiest macronutrient for the body to convert to energy because of their chemical makeup. When carbs are digested, they are turned quickly into glucose, which the body uses for energy. The body breaks these molecules down quicker than any other macronutrient. However, simplest does not mean "best." I used to think that, because carbohydrates were the easiest for the body to convert to energy, that it was best to give my body plenty of carbs. That may be good advice for athletes or people who need a lot of energy and need it now, but it's not really applicable to my situation and probably not to yours either.

A good deal of information on carb consumption is taken from advice to athletes. Take, for instance, the idea that before a workout you need to "load up on carbs" because they are converted to energy the quickest.

That may work for a professional athlete with 5 to 12 percent body fat, who burns as many calories in one day as a normal person would burn in a week; but carb loading is not good as general advice. A popular "protein bar" that is sold right in most workout facilities is full of sugar with a little bit of protein and very high in calories. Some people want to have one before and after they work out, thinking they need the energy. What we really need is to follow information to help us meet our Lose It Forever goals—not some professional athlete's goals. After doing a little research I discovered that the body will convert anything to energy if the body needs it; not just carbs but fats, proteins, or even bone and muscle in extreme situations.

That's where knowledge comes in. It's not a good idea to just blindly follow advice you hear or read on the Internet. You don't need a sugary "sports drink" or a protein shake after a workout—in fact, that is a bad idea. First of all, you will be nullifying the value of the workout because you'll have consumed more calories than you've burned. Second, the sports drink will just cause an insulin response that is unhealthy for your body (more about this in a minute). And third, those drinks and protein bars are mostly sugar, so they will keep you on the sugar addiction cycle—great for their business, but terrible for your health. I personally find it better to eat a snack of lean protein before a workout, like a tuna salad with a low-calorie dressing, precisely because the body takes longer to process it to energy than carbs. By not loading my body up with sugar, I force it to pull fat stores from my cells.

TYPES OF CARBS

All carbohydrates are not created equal, which is why I am not against all carbs—just most of them. And remember, one piece of advice does not fit everyone in the same way. Our bodies are all different. Our upbringings and lifestyles and physical makeups are different. Our relative addictions to carbohydrates, which have a lot to do with how we are raised, are different.

So when I tell you that carbohydrates affect my body negatively, I am not going to flat out tell you to ban all carbohydrates from your life.

Rather, I am going to explain how they negatively affect your health and allow you to figure out which carbohydrates you are comfortable with and which you will modify or substitute. If you practice Modification Not Starvation, you will eat carbs. You will get them in what I call "filler calories"; I'll explain that in a little bit. First, let's look at so-called good carbohydrates versus bad carbohydrates.

Typically, good carbs are considered to be complex carbs, such as whole grain bread and low starch vegetables such as green beans or broccoli. A whole grain bread is not refined or overly processed. Just because a bread is brown does not mean it is made with whole grains. A sprouted grain bread, which is not ground into flour when making the bread, has so many whole grains that the body actually burns extra calories during the digestion process. That's because complex carbs are harder to digest than simple carbs.

I'm actually very hesitant to label any carbs "good." Not because they are not good for you, but because of what we do to good carbs. I've noticed that every time I talk to my students about carbs such as whole grain bread, many people start thinking, "Great, I can have it with my peanut butter and jelly sandwich." And when I mention broccoli, people want to load it with melted high-calorie cheese. When people hear oatmeal, they douse it with butter and brown sugar. So how good are your good carbs now? We can take even a good carbohydrate and make it bad.

Bad carbohydrates are considered to be processed or refined carbohydrates such as white bread, chips, ice cream, cookies, soda pop, and sugar-laden foods. The reason they're so bad is because they cause your blood sugar to rise for two or three hours after ingestion and trigger an insulin response. After this burst of energy, there's a crash. The only way to really avoid that crash is to come back and eat more of those bad carbohydrates, causing another insulin episode. My bottom line is, you can eat some good carbohydrates and still lose weight, but we're staying away from bad carbs.

THE CARBOHYDRATE-INSULIN CONNECTION

I mentioned that loading up on bad carbs causes an insulin response in your blood. Insulin is the hormone we're most concerned with when discussing carbohydrates and diet. It is so important that I need to try to explain how it works in laymen's terms.

Hormones are chemical messengers produced by glands and other organs of the body. These messengers travel through the bloodstream and cause changes in specific cells and tissues. Hormones regulate all kinds of processes: growth, sexual development, reproduction, sleep, hunger, digestion, production of blood cells, and many other functions.

As soon as you put food into your mouth, your body goes to work to break the food down for use as energy. Your teeth, tongue, saliva, and esophagus all work to mash the food up and break it down. Food travels through your esophagus to your stomach, where bile is released to further break the food down. From the stomach, food that will be used for nutrients and energy gets passed to the small intestine, and waste goes to the large intestines to be discarded. From the small intestine, the nutrients and sugars are passed over to the bloodstream and the sugars are turned into glucose.

Your blood delivers the glucose to all the cells of your body, which use it as energy. As you can see, glucose has a very important purpose. Glucose cannot stay in the bloodstream. Prolonged high levels of glucose in the blood can cause damage to the kidneys and arteries, among other problems. So glucose/sugar needs to be removed from your bloodstream and stored in the cells as energy.

Insulin is the hormone that gives the cells instructions for taking it in and storing the blood sugar—as fat. When the pancreas detects an increase in glucose levels in the bloodstream after a meal, the pancreas releases insulin into the bloodstream to open up the cells.

The problem comes when we continually have too much glucose in our bloodstream. The pancreas will continue to release insulin to deal with the glucose, but over time, the pancreas can become exhausted and produce less and less insulin, failing to keep blood sugar levels stable. In other situations, the body's cells and tissues do not follow the instructions of the insulin being produced and will not absorb the glucose as they are supposed to, causing glucose levels in the blood to rise. A lack of insulin created by the pancreas or cells' lack of response to insulin both create a condition known as insulin resistance. This is dangerous, as it will not only affect your mood, causing it to swing perceptibly throughout the day, but high blood sugar levels can make you susceptible to type 2 diabetes. When glucose builds up in the blood instead of going into the cells, it leads to diabetes complications like damage to the kidneys, heart, and eyes, diabetic coma, heart attack, or stroke.

I'm not trying to scare you, but what I want you to see here is that sugar can be a poison to the body. You need to understand that too much sugar in the blood can have very bad effects. You have to manage the amount of sugar in the body if you're going to regulate the amount of insulin being produced.

Managing blood sugar and insulin will also help regulate your mood throughout the day. When you have a large amount of glucose in the bloodstream, you feel pumped up because the body uses it for energy right away. You feel like you've got tons of "get-up-and-go." But pretty soon the insulin is released and pulls that blood sugar out of the bloodstream and stores it in your cells.

Then you have that crash I talked about. You have a precipitous decline in the way you feel. You no longer have that same spark of energy. This is what happens if you have a high-carbohydrate lunch. You feel good until about an hour afterward. Then you want to take a nap—or have another sugary snack or coffee to get another quick jolt. Energy products are constantly being marketed to address this "2:30 p.m. drop in energy."

So our goal when it comes to carbohydrates is to keep our insulin and blood sugar levels even throughout the day. We don't want to have these ups and downs, these spikes and crashes. A closely related goal is to starve the cells of additional fuel (fat) and get the cells to release the fuel (fat) that is stored in them. Insulin is a storage hormone. Reduce your sugar and you can force the cells to release their fuel (fat) for the body to use as energy.

INTRODUCING THE FOUR CS

So how do we regulate the amount of glucose that gets into the blood at one time? The answer lies in considering the Four Cs. When we're practicing the principle of Modification Not Starvation, we need to have a correct understanding of carbohydrates.

CORRECT CALORIES, CAUTIOUS CARBS

The Four Cs means that we want to focus on counting calories with a cautious eye on carbohydrates.

The USDA has put forth a general macronutrient recommendation. It says that on a daily basis people should eat somewhere around:

55 percent carbohydrates
30 percent proteins
15 percent fats

When it comes to carbohydrates, their recommendation is not always exact—they suggest somewhere between 40 percent and 60 percent due to the fact that people process macronutrients differently. Of course, as you change the percentage of one macronutrient, the other percentages will change as well.

When the government released its food recommendations in the late 1970s, and then put them in pyramid form in 1992, those recommendations were very negative toward fat. It said that fat was bad, and that everybody in America should switch to more of a low-fat diet. Since that time, the obesity rate has skyrocketed. I believe that's because the food industry responded to the government and said, "Okay, we're going to follow these guidelines. However, flavor has to come from somewhere." So fat was taken out of food and sugar was put in. If you want to look at the real cause of American obesity over the past thirty years, I believe it is an incredible increase in the use of sugar.

Now don't go and start blaming your weight problems on the food industry or Uncle Sam. I'm just explaining why I think there is so much sugar in our processed foods. As I mentioned before, if we're going to Lose It Forever we need to take responsibility for our own health and not rely on anyone else. Nobody is making us eat fast food, processed food, and high-calorie food. We need to start forming good Forever Habits that take some of those ever-present carbohydrates out and replace them with something else. That's part of what I have done and I have seen great results from it.

One of the reasons I can help you be successful is because I don't just tell you what to eat, I try to educate you about nutrition so that you can make your own food choices. I went through this exact same process myself.

PETE'S PERSONALIZED CARBOHYDRATE RATIO

I practice a different macronutrient ratio than the one recommended by the USDA, and I want you to consider discovering your own as well. Here is mine:

15 percent carbohydrates
85 percent proteins and fats

I keep my carbs right around 15 percent of my Personalized Fuel Plan and my proteins and fats somewhere right around 85 percent. I discovered this quite by accident during my time on *The Biggest Loser* Ranch. I came in from Michigan to Simi Valley, California, and they had all of this beautiful California fruit lying around, so I would eat six or seven huge, luscious oranges a day thinking that would help me lose weight. They were delicious, but I noticed that I wasn't getting quite the same weight loss results as the other contestants, even though I was working out just as hard as everyone else and keeping my calories in line.

As an experiment, I cut back on the number of oranges I ate. At the same time, I started eating more proteins and fats as I ate fewer carbohydrates. While I did not change my overall caloric intake, just like that, my weight loss improved and I was able to lose weight much quicker. I discovered I lost weight with more consistency as I began to cut back on some of the carbohydrates, including the natural sugars found in fruit, and ate more proteins and fats. (I do consume some fruits; I just consume lower-sugar fruits such as strawberries and blueberries. I will talk about this a little bit more in Chapter 8 when we create our Perfect Personalized Forever Meal Plan.)

The reason I tell you this story about the oranges is because each one of us is slightly different in how our bodies process different foods. I'm explaining what macronutrient levels work best for me, but each of us must discover for ourselves what ratio works for us.

You can discover this, of course, as you're writing in your LIF2

Success Journal on a daily basis. You will notice those times when you feel sluggish, or those times when the food simply doesn't agree with you. If you go to a restaurant and have a high-carbohydrate lunch and within an hour you feel like you're crashing and you want to go to sleep, you must understand it's probably because of the extra carbohydrates you took in during lunch. Your journal will help you figure out what percentages make you feel most energetic. Remember, we want to watch calories but keep a cautious eye on carbs as well, which will result in Correct Calories, Cautious Carbs.

Once you have been journaling regularly you will have two great tools at your disposal—your Personal Daily Fuel Goal and your Personal Macronutrient Ratio. You should memorize them both.

THE OTHER GUYS

We talk a lot about carbohydrates, and rightly so, because they make up so much of our diets. But that's not the end of the story. As I said, I reduced my carbs and increased the other two macronutrients—protein and fat.

Proteins come from meat, of course, but also from dairy, beans, nuts, seeds, and some vegetables like spinach. Proteins are important for healthy cells and muscles, as well as the hormones that are the messengers of our bodies. And contrary to what some programs will tell you, you need fat in your diet as well. Unsaturated fat is best, in the form of nuts, fish, healthy oils like olive oil, and avocados. But I have a special place in my heart and house for lean burgers and steaks.

GOOD FAT—IS THERE SUCH A THING?

Research tells us that we need fats in our diet, pure and simple. We need fat to provide energy, to cushion organs, and help with growth and development. Fats are also great at meals because even though they contain more calories per gram than carbs, they are known to stimulate satiety, which means they make you feel fuller faster. Fats also don't cause an insulin response (as long as you're not combining them with carbs, of course), so as you replace some carbs with fats, you'll start getting off of the sugar addiction yo-yo.

Good fats are natural fats—think of fish, which contains omega-3 fatty acids, so they are very good. The monounsaturated—or liquid—fats, such as those found in nuts and olive oil, are very, very good.

Bad fats basically come down to man-made fats—commonly called trans fats. I am not anti-fat, but I am absolutely anti–trans fat. If you pay attention to health literature at all, you've read the many studies that talk about how bad trans fats are for your arteries and your heart. Companies are now revealing the trans fat content in their foods, so it's fairly easy to recognize them in your processed foods. Be aware, though, that a product can claim to be "trans fat–free" if it contains less than 0.5 gram of trans fat per serving. But have you seen the serving size of some of these foods? Who can eat five potato chips? It's easy to eat four or six servings, in which case we're getting too much trans fat. We want to stay away from these types of foods as much as possible. Once again, the main principle we want to remember here is to stay away from refined carbohydrates, which will keep us away from trans fats as well.

THE WHITE POISONS

As you modify the foods you like, pay special attention to the white poisons—sugar, salt, and refined flour (notice that two out of three are carbs). We talked a little bit about the dangers of salt at the beginning of the chapter, but salt can also affect weight loss. When I would struggle with losing pounds on the ranch, Jillian taught me to look at the salt content of my food. Salt is a weight loss killer. When you consume a lot of salt, your body retains more water as it seeks to dilute the excessive salt concentrations.

Whenever I have struggled with my weight loss, I would cut my salt intake to between 1200 to 1600 milligrams, while still eating very well, and the weight loss would fall right back in line.

We've already talked about sugar, too—it is addictive, it causes an insulin response within your body, and it can also cause certain types of food cravings. I've already expressed my opinion that the high sugar content of processed foods is helping to keep 60 percent of us overweight in the United States.

But there is one white poison I have not talked about yet in detail—refined flour.

HOW TO RUIN GOOD FOOD

We love to take our food and batter it, especially African Americans and folks from the South. Although this is a tasty tradition, it's terrible for your waistline.

I remember one time—before *The Biggest Loser*—I went to a little shrimp shack in Inkster, Michigan. This little dive could have been featured on one of those cable TV food shows like *Diners, Drive-ins and Dives*. It was only open three days a week—Friday, Saturday, and Sunday—and the line to get in stretched all the way around the building. After tasting the food, I understood why. The cooks dipped the shrimp in batter and fried each piece. Then they took the fried shrimp, dipped it in batter for a second time, and fried each piece again!

So the cooks would take a rather small, bland piece of shrimp and batter it up so much that it quadrupled in size and was no longer recognizable as the food it started out as. But like lots of other people who stood in line to eat it, I absolutely loved it.

Frying is an incredibly bad way to treat my waistline and my blood sugar, but it's an amazing way to treat my palate! So this is what we want to be aware of when it comes to flour. The body looks at flour as a carbohydrate, so there's an insulin response that happens, followed by a perceptible energy crash. Not only that, but by adding flour and frying the food in oil, you're adding tons of calories that you don't need. You probably won't be able to avoid the white poisons completely, but replacing them whenever possible will get you marching toward losing it forever.

ENERGY TO BURN

I mentioned thermogenesis—which involves burning calories to digest your food—in Chapter 5. If you change your macronutrient ratios—meaning the ratio of carbohydrates, fats, and proteins you eat—you can change the amount of energy needed to digest and store your food. You can burn more calories simply by eating more of one type of food and less of another, because certain foods are easier for your body to process than others. Easier means your body doesn't have to work as hard, so you don't burn as many calories in the digestive process.

If you're a typical American, your diet is high in processed foods and fast food. You could switch to a higher protein diet, lower in refined carbs and high in whole grains, low-starch vegetables, and low-sugar fruits. In so doing, you could easily burn a few extra calories each and every day, not to mention that you'd feel better, think more clearly, and probably lose some weight.

I advocate creating your own Perfect Personalized Fuel Plan because you're going to make what you eat—and how you eat it—fit into your busy life. You can get full, eat cleaner, stay within your calories, reduce your carbohydrates, lower your sugar intake, and generally enjoy life as you lose that next Forever Five.

KEY POINTS

- We need to understand and practice the Four Cs: Correct Calories, Cautious Carbs.
- Each of us must discover for ourselves what carbohydrate ratio works for us.
- As you modify the foods you like, pay special attention to the white poisons—sugar, salt, and refined flour (notice that two out of three are carbs).
- If we change our macronutrient ratios—meaning the ratio of carbohydrates, fats, and proteins we eat—we can change the amount of energy needed to digest and store our food. Although this is not our main focus, as we burn most of our calories through exercise, it does make a difference.

CHAPTER 7 CHALLENGES

New Challenges | Adjust Your Macronutrient Ratio

We can actually eat more food with fewer calories by swapping certain types of foods with others. For instance, try swapping out high-calorie carbs with lower-calorie vegetables.

Ongoing Challenges | Continue Your Food Journal

Continue to write in your food journal. Pay special attention to your body's reaction to various carbohydrate ratios so you can adjust them if necessary. Write down your modifications to the white poisons as you come up with them.

Trumpet Your Forever Habit Formed

As you form Forever Habits one at a time, celebrate by commenting at www.PeteThomas.com. Read the posts of others who've achieved their goal and share your own success.

"My husband and I had been trying to lose weight for over twenty years, unsuccessfully. We actually made a pact about not telling anybody that we were taking LIF2. I guess that was our fallback plan in case it didn't work. After a short time, we miraculously started seeing changes, so we could see that it was actually working, and we started getting excited about it. I've lost 60 pounds so far, and my husband has lost 75. We now have the knowledge that will help to maintain our goal weights. It can't be taken away. We don't ever have to be as we once were."

—CARMEN, LIF2 STUDENT

CHAPTER

PREPARING FOR YOUR PERFECT PERSONALIZED FOREVER MEAL PLAN

BEFORE I WENT TO *THE BIGGEST LOSER*, I ATTENDED A CONFERENCE hosted by The Potter's House Church in Dallas, Texas. At the time I was close to 400 pounds and extremely unhealthy. One day I went out on Jet Skis on the lake with a buddy of mine. I fell off my Jet Ski and could not get back on. I tried and tried for thirty minutes but could not pull myself back up. Every time I tried to pull myself up on the back of the Jet Ski, the front of it would pop up and I would not be able get on. My buddy tried valiantly to help me, and tried to offset my weight by standing on the front of the Jet Ski, but he ended up falling in the water himself. After all that struggling I was completely out of breath and had no energy left in my body. The rental company had to come out and tow my rig back to shore with me holding on to the back of it. It seemed like it took forever to be pulled back to shore, and I felt like I was about to slip off and drown at any moment.

Lesson of the story? Your extra weight will kill you. You have an opportunity to rescue yourself if you can change the way you live and keep living that way. In this chapter I want to guide you through the process of creating your own Perfect Personalized Forever Meal Plan. Halfway through you're going to say to yourself, "This is a lot of work." You're right, it is going to take some time. But remember that you are worth it. Your health is worth it. Helping those around you is worth it. So take the time to develop some new Forever Habits as we continue our journey toward losing that extra weight.

THE BEST OF BOTH WORLDS

The primary reason that my students (and I) Lose It Forever is that this program incorporates the best of both "diet plan" worlds. That means that we will be taking advantage of the best aspects of both counting and set plans. We're going to incorporate the variety of a counting plan (in which you can eat anything you want as long as it is within caloric limits) and the discipline of a set plan (repeating our favorite nutritious foods over and over to keep us within our goals).

I've said this before, but it bears repeating: Losing weight is not our goal; learning to eat correctly for the rest of our lives is the real goal. To do this we will develop our own Perfect Personalized Forever Meal Plan.

We will need both discipline and variety to make this program work. I consider myself fairly disciplined in many areas of my life, but obviously I struggle when it comes to my eating habits. Because of this lack of discipline, I can't keep eating the same thing each and every day. However, I can eat the same thing week in and week out. If I can incorporate a little bit more variety in my week, the food selections stay interesting, so I don't get bored and binge just to get some different flavors. So variety really will help you stay disciplined. That's the goal of our menu plan.

Our ultimate goal is to create a menu plan that allows us to follow it faithfully. If you can stick to your meal plan on a regular basis, then you are going to be successful long-term. But that requires that you have enough variety in there to keep you happy.

Before we develop our meal plan, we have to answer some critical questions, like when do I eat, where should I eat, what should I eat, and so on. When I set out to live a healthy life and stay thin, I found answers to those questions. You will answer them, too.

Before you get to that, though, it's helpful to understand some basic things about metabolism and hormones. This will give you an understanding of the cravings and struggles with food that we all have. When I began to research these concepts after my time on *The Biggest Loser*, I really got an understanding of how my body works and why I have certain struggles with foods at certain times of the day. This learning is an essential first step in developing a Perfect Personalized Forever Meal Plan.

We're going to talk about some of the hormones that affect how you eat, so that you'll know more about how your body works. I'm not a fan of programs that just tell you what to eat and when—I want you to be educated so that you can make lifelong changes to your health. Anyone can tell you "what" to eat, but if you understand "why" you should eat a certain thing at a certain time, you will begin to develop Forever Habits. I'll illustrate what I mean in the next section.

HORMONES—THE BODY'S MESSENGERS

Last chapter, we talked about insulin, an important hormone in regulating blood sugar. Hormones are chemical messengers produced by glands and other organs of the body. These messengers travel through the bloodstream and cause changes in specific cells and tissues. Hormones regulate all kinds of processes: growth, sexual development, reproduction, sleep, hair growth, hunger, digestion, production of blood cells, and many other functions.

For simplicity, I'm going to categorize the hormones as "good" hormones and "bad" hormones as they concern weight loss. Of course, every hormone has a purpose, so there's really no such thing as a bad hormone. But when it comes to weight loss, some hormones are better than others. So we need to understand how a few of these chemical messengers affect weight loss when we're putting together our nutrition plan, because that will determine, for instance, what times of day we're going to eat.

"GOOD" HORMONES

HGH, or human growth hormone, stimulates the building of bones and muscles. It is responsible primarily for growth in children. But this hormone can also assist with weight loss by causing the body to use fat stores for energy. HGH is typically released at night. The bad news is that it can also be blocked from being released when refined carbohydrates are present after a certain time of the night. When I realized the role of this hormone, I decided to be more careful about what I eat late at night. I have a snack, but it's not ice cream and cake like it used to be before I went on *The Biggest Loser*. Now I'll have something lower in calories and sugar like sugar-free Jell-O or low-fat string cheese.

The next hormone is leptin, which brings messages to the brain. I call this a good hormone because it signals the brain that you've had enough to eat. Leptin can decrease our appetite, as well as cause an increase in metabolism. Metabolism refers to the process of converting the fuel in our food into the energy we need to live. Interestingly, obese people have been found to be resistant to this hormone. The good news is that you can turn that resistance around by losing weight and exercising. I told you before that for a long time I did not obey my "stop" signal when my stomach was full. Now that I've lost a bunch of weight, this chemical messenger is free to do its job—and I obey the message.

We have two hormones that work together to build muscle and regulate reproduction, development, and overall heath—testosterone and estrogen. Men produce more testosterone than estrogen, and women produce the opposite. The amount and source of estrogen production, either from the ovaries, from the liver, or from fat tissue, greatly affect obesity, metabolism, and disease. For men, low testosterone levels are often treated with an increase in exercise and accelerated weight loss. In short, exercise and proper nutrition are essential for the proper production and regulation of both of these essential hormones.

You should also know something about serotonin and endorphins. These hormones give us a happy feeling. They've been called God's natural antidepressants because they give us a natural high. They are released during and after exercise. You may have heard about the runner's high;

that refers to the release of serotonin and endorphins into the bloodstream after a long run. It's an amazing feeling to have an intense workout and then feel awesome about yourself. So if you are depressed about life, God has already given you a way to deal with that feeling. It's not drugs. It's not alcohol. It's not sugar. It's exercise. Good, hard, intense exercise releases these endorphins, and you just magically feel better about yourself. Knowing about the release of these hormones has helped me change how I deal with stress—I have turned from food to exercise. It has made a big difference in my health and my psychological well-being.

"BAD" HORMONES

Now I want to talk about one of the bad hormones—ghrelin. This is what I call a time-released hormone, and it is primarily responsible for signaling hunger and slowing metabolism. It responds to emotional and physical stress. Some studies have shown that ghrelin will signal the body that you are hungry at certain times of the day, even if you've just eaten. This is important information, because if you've just gone to lunch at 1:00, and at 2:00 like clockwork your body tells you you're hungry—that is probably a sign that ghrelin is sending a message.

One particular program calls this hormonal signal "head hunger," which is a good name. If you're used to eating at 2:00 every day, then one day you eat at 1:00, ghrelin is going to signal you at 2:00 that "Hey, it's time to eat" even though you don't need any food. It's also known as a stress hormone or a "fight or flight" hormone. You have to be really careful about responding to these signals in a healthy way. That's why I wanted to include this section on hormones—so that you can be educated on how they affect your weight loss efforts. The next time you "feel" hungry, assess whether it is head hunger or stomach hunger by evaluating the time and type of your last meal as well as you current stress levels.

The next hormone I want to talk about is cortisol. It's a physical and emotional stress-release hormone that can contribute to weight gain. It does this by increasing our appetite, blood pressure, and blood sugar when calories are restricted below recommended levels.

Remember in Chapter 5 I mentioned that women should never eat below 1200 calories and men should never eat below 1600 calories daily?

This is why. When we eat too little food, our bodies go into something called starvation mode. Starvation mode involves the release of cortisol into the body, which causes the body to hold on to fat stores and, in rare instances, even utilize bone and muscle for fuel instead of that fat. So you want to be careful about consuming too few calories. Believe it or not, eating too few calories is really bad for your weight loss efforts.

INSULIN

Insulin is absolutely the most important hormone to be concerned with when trying to lose weight and stay healthy. We already talked about insulin in Chapter 7, but I want to restate the main idea because it affects what you'll put into your Perfect Personalized Forever Meal Plan.

Insulin is released when glucose enters the bloodstream. The glucose comes from carbohydrates that your digestive system has broken down. Insulin is like a key that unlocks the cells, allowing them to absorb the glucose for energy. Our goal is to keep our blood sugar level even throughout the day so that we don't get peaks of energy and then valleys of sluggishness. You can keep your blood sugar level constant by building a good Perfect Personalized Forever Meal Plan and sticking to it faithfully.

YOU MUST E.A.N. YOUR WEIGHT LOSS

So how does all this knowledge play into our weight loss journey? Once you have an understanding of these hormones, then you can more readily answer some common questions:

- How often should I personally eat?
- When should I personally eat?
- Where should I personally eat?
- What should I personally eat?
- How do I personally shop for food to eat?

Once answered, all of these questions will lead us to creating our Perfect Personalized Weekly Food Menu, the twin to our Perfect Personalized Forever Meal Plan.

When it comes to weight loss, I've coined an expression to help guide myself in some of these things. I have come to recognize that I have to E.R.N. my weight loss. E.R.N. stands for exercise, rest, and nutrition. And hormones play a large role in each of these elements.

- **Exercise** can cause us to lose weight because it burns up calories and at the same time increases our metabolism, while relieving stress through the release of serotonin and endorphins.
- **Rest** allows the body to recover and rebuild itself through the release of good hormones.
- **Nutrition** fuels the body's daily activities; when done correctly, good nutrition helps keep blood sugar levels even, which helps regulate hormones and controls our appetite.

Determining how often you eat is very important. No single answer works for everybody, but I tell my students that they should try to eat at least three times a day depending on their Personal Daily Fuel Goal. What you really need to be successful in losing it forever is a Personalized Meal Plan based upon your own Personal Daily Fuel Goal and lifestyle. This is not as complicated as it sounds—we'll do it together in the next section.

YOUR PERFECT PERSONALIZED FOREVER MEAL PLAN

One of my students told me about her eating habits. She said, "I've been eating good during the day, but at night I have been really struggling. I often eat 1500 or 1600 calories at dinner alone, regardless of what I've eaten during the day." She was small in stature and she understood that having so many calories at dinner was not good for her weight loss goal. I told her, "You need to adjust your eating throughout the day, if your schedule allows it, so that you're not overeating at night." She began to eat several times a day, which caused her to pay closer attention to what she was eating, and she started to see the scale move again.

I often tell the story of the gentleman who lost approximately 30 pounds just by planning a snack into his day. This man would eat three meals a day religiously. When he came home from work, he would eat dinner at 5:30 every day. Then somewhere around 8:30 p.m. he would be hungry again, so he would have dessert. He struggled to lose those last 30 pounds that he was looking for.

To combat the negative aspects of this routine, he started a new Forever Habit. When he came home from work at 5:30, he began making himself a snack consisting of low-fat cottage cheese with a couple of peach slices. That snack would hold him perfectly fine until he started eating dinner around 7:00 p.m. After that, he would no longer eat his dessert at 8:30 because he was still full. He did this for about three months and he lost nearly a pound every three days for a total of about 30 pounds. It worked because he had effectively pushed his dessert right off the cliff, which helped him stay within his calorie budget.

That menu and plan worked for him because it worked within his Personal Daily Fuel Goal and his schedule. That being said, we now have to figure out how many times a day you are going to eat.

FIRST THE BASICS . . . WHEN SHOULD I EAT?

The main purpose of figuring out how many times you're going to eat is so that you can maintain your energy level by maintaining stable blood sugar levels. And as I've said before, this is going to be dependent on your lifestyle and on your Personal Daily Fuel Goal. Let me use another example.

Let's say that your Personal Daily Fuel Goal is 1600 calories a day, and you decide that you're going to have six meals a day. Well, that comes out to right around 266 calories per meal. Now personally, I would find it very hard to eat a good meal for 266 calories. It's more realistic to have four meals of 400 calories each. That's a little bit better to work with. Another option would be to have three meals of 400 calories each, plus two 200-calorie snacks. That sounds a little more doable.

Your meal plan also has to fit in with your work schedule. Say you're the ultrafocused type of worker, and you just dive into your work without spending a lot of time thinking about food until the day is over. Then at night you're scarfing down 1600 calories at dinner. That is not really healthy. We want to make sure that you space your meals out a little bit so that you're not overloading your system with one large meal.

You can see that the question of how often you eat is going to depend on you as an individual. This is where our plan is different. You have to design the details of this plan yourself. If you think about this, it makes absolute sense. After all, every one of you reading this book has different schedules, habits, and responsibilities. There is no one-size-fits-all program that fits every lifestyle. The best thing to do is to take the good, solid guidelines contained in this plan and customize them to your own needs.

Before being cast on *The Biggest Loser*, I attempted a plan that required that I eat six to eight times a day. At the time my business caused me to travel across the Detroit metro area and consult with clients on their information technology projects. I would pack up my grilled chicken breasts in the morning and head out on my way in the summer heat. By lunchtime my well-prepared chicken would invariably have a lovely green fuzz developing on it from sitting in the car while I was in client meetings. And it did not taste like guacamole. As a precaution I would microwave the chicken—and pray—so that I did not get sick. Needless to say, this plan did not work for my circumstances without some substantial modifications.

Not only did this plan not work for me, but I eventually learned that plans requiring six to eight meals a day were popularized by bodybuilders who needed to consume between 3000 and 5000 "clean" calories over the course of the day in order to gain weight and build muscle mass. Needless to say, I am not intentionally trying to hit either of those goals. The knowledge of how this particular method came into popularity caused me to reconsider everything I read about exercise and nutrition.

I have now learned to look at everything I read with a new set of eyes and a healthy skepticism. When I read anything about exercise and nutrition, I ask myself four basic questions:

1. What is the author's intention or reason for writing? To persuade? To compare and analyze? To criticize?
2. Is there any bias or motivation on behalf of the author? In other words, is the author trying to sell me something? Or does he need to reach a certain conclusion to continue grant funding?

3. What is the opposite argument or opinion?
4. Does this information apply to me and my situation? For example, is this information written for professional athletes or people who run fifty miles a week?

That's why Lose It Fast, Lose It Forever is different. There is no "one-size-fits-all" answer here. I will tell you specifically what to eat in Step 3 so that you can Lose It Fast, but to Lose It Forever, you have to answer the question "What is my plan?" For me personally, I eat somewhere right around three or four meals a day at 400 to 500 calories each. That is what works for me, with a couple of snacks included. Together we will figure out your Forever Plan.

A GOOD BEGINNING—EATING BREAKFAST

Now that you've figured out how often to eat, I'm sure your next question is "When should I eat?" The first thing I want you to understand is that you must eat breakfast each and every day. As a general rule—and I do mean *rule*—you need to eat within the first thirty minutes of getting up.

If you're like me and you like to get up and immediately go out the door for a jog, then you'll stretch that time to within the first ninety minutes of getting up. But the fact of the matter is, you need to shove down some food for the sake of your metabolism. If you're out the door and you're having breakfast at work several hours after you've awakened, then that's not breakfast. Breakfast literally means to break the fast, and in this case, the fast was the time you were sleeping. Even though it's in the morning, if you're not eating within thirty minutes of when you wake up, that's not breakfast.

I was being interviewed on the radio one morning, and the host told me about his insanely early schedule. He would get up at 3:00 in the morning, get himself ready, and come into work. He would get on the air at 6:00 a.m., so he would have a bite to eat right around 8:00 in the morning—a good five hours after he woke up. He claimed he was having breakfast because he ate it "at breakfast time." I said, "No, that's actually pretty bad. You are not having breakfast. You've been up for five hours—you're having what really amounts to more of a lunch." Guess what—this guy struggled with his weight, too.

The purpose of breakfast is twofold. First, it's to start up your metabolism and let the body know that food is coming. It's announcing to the body, "Do not release bad hormones! I'm not going to put you in starvation mode." It gets the body burning calories through the digestive process, which we discussed earlier. The second purpose of breakfast is to get you to the next meal without being unnecessarily hungry. If you eat breakfast and you're hungry within an hour of eating, then you need to tweak the components of that breakfast to create satisfaction and satiety. You may need to add more fillers to your breakfast or even add fat to your breakfast for satiety. A good breakfast will start your metabolic engine and help get you to your next fuel stop without any undue stops by the vending machine.

This is very important—you don't necessarily have to eat breakfast-type foods. Who said that eggs have to be your breakfast food? Who says that you have to have bacon or whole grain toast? You can eat some of the food that you have left over from dinner from the night before if you want. I've heard people say, "I just don't have time to make breakfast in the morning." The truth is, you're not *making* the time. Take some food from dinner the night before if you need to, or make breakfast on the weekends for the entire week. Just make sure that whatever you eat, you have something at breakfast time.

A GOOD ENDING—THE LAST MEAL OF THE DAY

When it comes to dinner, a common recommendation is to have your last meal of the day three to four hours before bedtime. Any more than that and you may be hungry right before you go to bed, so you'll be tempted to have an unhealthy snack. If you eat dinner much less than three to four hours before, you may not give your body time to digest it before you hit the hay. The key, as always, is to experiment and find what works best for you.

I get asked quite often about snacking late at night. You've probably heard of studies that claim late-night eating causes weight gain. That's true, but that statement doesn't give you the entire story. Think about it: If you were to have steamed broccoli every night at 10:30 p.m., do you really think you'd gain all kinds of extra weight? It's unlikely.

The truth of the matter is that these studies are done with people who have already nearly overeaten throughout the day. If you're staying within your calories, food at the end of the day is not harmful in and of itself. But you do have to watch out for refined carbohydrates. Refined carbohydrates block the release of hormones that help the body burn fat. And you certainly can't burn fat when you're sleeping and not moving around. That's why I avoid refined carbohydrates late at night.

Actually, I watch out for refined carbohydrates any time of the day. Watch out for the cookies, the cakes, the snacks, and all of those different things. I told you earlier about my typical Friday night. Not only was I overeating, but I was consuming bad carbs late at night. That type of eating can reverse any gains you made during the week on your quest toward losing those pounds forever.

The bottom line is, even with my rules about a good beginning and a good ending, we have to remember that this is personal. You have to figure out what works for you. For example, I know two people who eat one meal a day and are in incredible physical condition. They both work out super-consistently and have done so for more than three decades. If you're overweight, then that particular plan will not be for you; you probably will need to eat throughout the day.

WHERE SHOULD I EAT?

Because this plan is so flexible, we can really eat anywhere we want. With one exception: It would be best to avoid eating in your car, even if you are forced to eat fast food. Do not go through the drive-through; go into the fast-food restaurant to slow down the eating process. Take your time ordering your food and then sit down and eat. After you sit, slow down your eating. This should actually cause you to think about what you're doing and maybe even allow you to enjoy your food a little bit more. When I eat while driving, I seldom enjoy the taste of the food and rarely am I aware of how much I am eating.

Similar principles can also be applied to eating at home. Some people call it "mindful eating." If you are so busy that you have to fix quick, high-calorie food for dinner, you will not be helping yourself lose weight. Take time to prepare healthy food. Turn it into relationship-building time by involving your family in the preparation. When you eat, slow down. Put down your fork between bites so that you'll savor the taste and give yourself a chance to feel full when you are full.

Be careful of eating in front of the TV. One study demonstrated that people who munch mindlessly in front of the TV consume 20 to 60 percent more than if they pay attention to what they're eating. Stick to your planned snacks, even in front of the TV. This is another Forever Habit that will keep you healthy long after you've lost the weight you want to lose.

WHAT SHOULD I EAT?

Meal planning essentially comes down to laying out a menu that keeps you within your Personal Daily Fuel Goal yet provides enough variety to keep you from feeling like you're "dieting." To really keep you happy, each and every meal must have three critical components. I call these components "The Three Fs."

INTRODUCING PETE'S MEAL PLANNING SUCCESS SECRET—THE THREE FS

Every single meal in our meal plan needs to have three things: a fluid, a filler, and a feast. You've probably noticed that I like to use alliteration because it helps me remember things. For instance, many people already have a "fluid" with their meal, but this will remind us that the drink does not get a free pass—it has to be lower calorie, too. To properly plan a meal we will use these Three Fs as a guide. A fluid will be a zero- or low-calorie drink. A filler will consist of soups, salads, and vegetables that will add bulk to your stomach and help fill you up. The feast is the actual main dish that we look forward to eating.

For example, let's say I am planning on going to a steakhouse to eat. What would I really be looking forward to eating at a steakhouse? An amazing steak! And that is the case if I am going to a great fish place or cooking at home. I look to enjoy the feast and save the bulk of calories on all the other dishes.

Here are some examples of the Three Fs:

FLUID

- Water or zero-calorie flavored water
- Green tea or tea with sugar substitute
- Diet soda or Crystal Light

FILLER

- Low-calorie soups—like Progresso Light or a low-fat broth-based soup. Soups decrease hunger and are a staple filler on our plan.
- Large salad—I am a member of the More Food Family (more about the Food Families in a minute), so I use lots of low-calorie ingredients such as lettuce, cut-up red/yellow/green bell peppers, cherry or grape tomatoes, onions, garlic cloves, cucumbers, sliced jalapeño peppers, banana pepper rings, mushrooms, sunflower seeds, shredded red cabbage, just a few raisins, sliced sweet pickles, and black and green olives. I also use low-calorie dressing such as low-fat Italian. I typically use very little or no cheese, eggs, or bacon toppings in order to keep the calories low.
- Low-starch vegetables—The key to eating and enjoying vegetables is in the preparation. Many of our parents may have severely overcooked vegetables, so we never discovered their amazing taste. Then we load our vegetables with cheese and butter and other toppings until we no longer taste the actual flavor. I make sure my vegetables are prepared in a way that does not add calories, such as by steaming, baking, grilling, and sautéing without oil. I use some or all of the following vegetables: spinach, (collard, turnip, and mustard) greens, cabbage, mushrooms, asparagus, green beans, broccoli, cauliflower, green or red bell peppers, jalapeño peppers, summer squash, zucchini, green onions, Brussels sprouts, alfalfa or bean sprouts, snow peas, tomatoes, water chestnuts, kale, bok choy, celery, eggplant, tomatillos, artichokes, radishes, sea vegetables, turnips, leeks, pumpkin, fennel, okra, celery. I also add

avocado, which technically is a fruit, but is also a healthy fat and helps keep me full.

■ As you season your fillers and feasts, look for these condiments, spices, and supplies: garlic, black pepper, basil, curry powder, turmeric, chili powder, crushed red pepper, dill, cinnamon, rosemary, parsley, salt-free spice blends, allspice, mustard, reduced-sugar ketchup, light or low-fat salad dressing, balsamic vinegar, lemon juice, low-sugar pasta sauce, hot sauce, salsa, low-sodium beef and chicken broth, and non-stick cooking spray.

FEAST

I am a meat guy. I enjoy meats of every type. Preparation and selection is key. I prepare my food by baking, grilling, or broiling. I select meats that are lean or lower in fat. Some of my favorite lean meats include pork loin, tenderloin, lean pork chops, chicken, turkey, lean chicken or turkey burgers, lean chicken or turkey sausages, Canadian bacon, low-fat or fat-free lunch meats (such as turkey from the deli), 96% lean ground beef, lean steaks such as sirloin, short loin, top loin, and tri-tip, as well as seafood such as shrimp, lobster, whitefish, salmon, tilapia, and tuna.

Some of your feasts are going to contain or be accompanied by dairy, breads, and grains. I look for low-carb tortillas, light whole grain bread and buns, sprouted grain bread, quinoa, steel-cut oatmeal, low-fat or reduced-fat cheese, egg substitutes, and egg whites.

If meat isn't your thing, you will still have a "feast." It would simply be your main dish. The most effective way to modify your feast is to substitute lower-calorie vegetables from the list above in place of some of the higher calorie meats or pastas. This will allow you to eat the same weight, or volume of food, but you will be filling up on food that has fewer calories. For example, if you love pizza, try making it a thin-crust pizza with lower-calorie cheese; instead of high-calorie pepperoni, substitute turkey pepperoni and then load it up with generous helpings of onions, bell peppers, mushrooms, olives, tomatoes, and any other vegetables that sound good to you. You won't feel deprived because you're eating a lot of volume, and it will taste great. Or take your lasagna and substitute fat-free ricotta cheese for regular cheese, then load up the dish with lean ground turkey or lean hamburger, as well as spinach, squash, zucchini, and onions.

BONUS—FUN FUEL

For little after-dinner snacks I avoid high-sugar pies and cakes by having my own selection of low-calorie snacks and fruits. They include fat-free Cool Whip, fat-free Reddi-wip, sugar-free Popsicles, no-sugar-added Fudgsicles, sugar-free Jell-O, carb-control and low-calorie yogurts, pickles, and light Laughing Cow cheese. Also look for fruits that are lower in sugar such as raspberries, blackberries, strawberries, blueberries, apples, watermelon, cantaloupe, honeydew, grapefruit, rhubarb, and cranberries. (There is some disagreement about what constitutes a low- or high-sugar fruit, but these are the ones I stick to.)

Let me give you another example from my own life. Breakfast is not typically the best time for me to have a lot of variety, so I get up and scarf down the same thing day after day. It's mostly due to a lack of time. For breakfast I have:

- Fluid—32 ounces of Crystal Light Classic Orange
- Filler—four servings of Egg Beaters with some I Can't Believe It's Not Butter! spray on it
- Feast—nine slices of turkey bacon

The feast is that item that you really enjoy. For my breakfast, it is turkey bacon every day.

I typically have much more variety in my own meal plan when it comes to lunch and dinner. At lunch I'm going to have my fluid, typically 32 ounces of water or Diet Sunkist. Then I'm going to have my filler, which is a salad with low-calorie salad dressing every day. Typically my feast is some type of sandwich. If I'm making a sandwich, I'm making it using a low-carb tortilla wrap, some tomatoes, and light Miracle Whip. The type of sandwich changes from day to day to provide variety. My dinners vary even more than this. You can see a complete rundown of my weekly meal plan later in this section.

To avoid feeling like you're starving yourself, every meal needs to contain your version of a feast. This will keep you from that feeling of being deprived. And to supplement your filler, get creative—throw everything you can into your salads, as I mentioned before. I typically go light on the cheese, because I want to keep the calories down. Cheese on my salad is negotiable, so I save those calories for my feast.

The meal plan I've sketched out for you is based on a really basic "three main meals a day" model. If you decide to eat more than three times a day, as I often do, you've got a couple of different options. I'll plan out seven different things that I'm going to eat for snacks, or I take my meals and make them a little larger, then cut them up and save them to eat later. If you want to, you can make a really large dinner and divide it up into two or three different meals.

PETE'S WEEKLY MENU—EXAMPLE

I list my regular weekly menu here as a way of showing you how I actually put together my food choices on a weekly basis. You also will be planning out your own weekly food menu to help you stay on track with your eating. Notice the Three Fs at every meal. Although my fluid and my filler look like they are similar at every meal, there is a lot of variety within those categories. As you build your menu, you could include even more variety; for instance, you could drink tea with a sugar substitute, zero-calorie flavored water, and so on.

PETE'S WEEKLY MEAL PLAN—LUNCH

	Fluid	Filler	Feast
Monday	32 ounces of water or diet soda	Large salad with added vegetables and low-calorie dressing, and/or soup	2 Whopper Jr. with extra everything, mustard, no bun, no mayo
Tuesday			Ham sandwich on a low-carb tortilla wrap, tomatoes, Miracle Whip Light
Wednesday			Turkey breast sandwich on a low-carb tortilla wrap, tomatoes, Miracle Whip Light
Thursday			Tuna sandwich on a low-carb tortilla wrap, tomatoes, Miracle Whip Light
Friday			Turkey hot dog with mustard, relish, Miracle Whip Light, no bun
Saturday			Teriyaki chicken wings (frozen, bought at supermarket)
Sunday			(I skip this meal on Sunday because of church and have an early dinner)

PETE'S WEEKLY MEAL PLAN—DINNER

	Fluid	Filler	Feast
Monday	32 ounces water or diet soda	Large salad with added vegetables and low-calorie dressing, and/or soup	Spinach, 96% lean hamburger
Tuesday			Green beans, chicken
Wednesday			Mashed cauliflower, pork loin
Thursday			Frozen veggie mix, seafood
Friday			Green beans, stir-fried leftovers
Saturday			Lima beans, turkey
Sunday			Mixed vegetables, mashed cauliflower, steak

BUT, PETE—YOU DIDN'T MENTION FIBER . . . WHAT ABOUT THE FIBER?

You hear a lot about fiber, that it keeps you feeling full longer, that it helps with digestion, and many other benefits. Many of these are good, but I personally believe that the focus on fiber misses the fact that people who struggle with food take good things and mess them up. If I take a piece of whole grain bread and add peanut butter and jelly, then I am adding a huge amount of calories to my fiber and diminishing any benefits. The same thing can be said of your morning whole grain muffin with butter or sour cream. There are just very few benefits left after we include all the extras we've been taught to add. By thinking in terms of filler, we naturally get the fiber in our diet through salads, soups, and vegetables. Don't believe me? You can simply do like the pharmacist who took one of my classes and calculated all the fiber in the fillers on my sample weekly menu. You will conclude, like she did, that we are getting more than enough fiber on this plan.

So as we begin to plan our weekly menus, we want to keep in mind some general guidelines:

- Eat four to six times a day depending on your Personal Daily Fuel Goal and work schedule.
- Don't fast for longer than twelve hours at a time.
- Make sure you eat a good breakfast.
- Eat clean at the end of the day and avoid refined carbohydrates.

YOUR MEAL PLAN

I want you to write down what your plan is (not your menu—that comes next). We have been tracking our calories day in and day out. We've been writing down everything we eat and how we feel. By now we should be able to figure out what is going to work best for us as we change the way we approach our food. Write it down in your LIF2 Success Journal or make a spreadsheet that includes the following:

- How often should I personally eat?
- When should I personally eat?
- Where should I personally eat?
- What should I personally eat?
- How do I personally shop for food to eat?

Now that you have sort of an outline of how you're going to approach your meals in the coming months, let me put one more piece of the puzzle into place. Then we'll finally write down our Perfect Personalized Forever Meal Plan.

INTRODUCING THE FOOD FAMILIES

Most of us fall into one of three "Food Families." No one really knows why we relate to food as we do; some of it is a result of genetics. But I believe a lot of it is how we were raised as well. For example, I grew up transient and was in and out of foster homes due to my mother's struggle with mental illness. When I was living with my mother, we experienced homelessness on more than one occasion. At other times, I would literally eat nothing but fast food for weeks on end, until my mother's money ran out. Then we would go without food for periods in which she convinced me we were fasting.

As a result of my upbringing, I never looked at food in its correct light, as fuel. Instead my taste buds were treated to the worst of both worlds. First, my taste buds became highly attuned to processed foods, with their lethal combination of fats, sugars, and refined flour. As you know, these are staples in fast-food restaurants. But more than that, I was always worried about not having enough food. Food for me was always more about availability than nutrition. That's why the amount of food I eat has always been foremost in my mind.

IN WHICH FOOD FAMILY DO YOU BELONG?

So what are these "Food Families"? In my personal observation and research, I have discovered that people fall into one of these families based on their attitude toward food and eating habits. While the principles in this program will help members of all three groups lose weight, each group will apply them in a little different way.

Food Is Fuel Family

People with a "normal" relationship with food fall into the Food Is Fuel Family. Without consciously identifying it this way, they simply look at food as the fuel necessary to get them through the day. Like a car filling up with gasoline, they eat just enough at one meal to last them until the next meal or fill-up. People in this family can get up and leave the table with food still on their plate because they feel satisfied. "Fuel" people don't like to feel overly full, and so avoid the feeling by eating moderately most of the time—even foods that they really like. I wish I was a member of this family. If I had been, I might never have struggled with extra weight.

Most people that struggle with food, while not having had the awkward upbringing that I had, tend to fall into one of the other food families: the More Food Family or the More Flavor Family.

More Food Family

For a large segment of the population, including many of the obese and super-obese, the amount of food consumed is very important. Often it is of prime importance. For better or worse, I include myself in this group. We are compulsive eaters, and many of us have an actual food addiction. When we sit down to eat, we consume as much as we can—even foods that we don't care for that much. Many of us in this family have certain "trigger" foods—specific foods that cause us to overeat because we just lose control. For the More Food Family to make a change in our eating, it is important to first have alternatives to our current eating habits as they relate to food choices and the amount of food.

More Flavor Family

For some people, the amount is not as important as flavor. I call these folk the More Flavor Family. For them, every bite or every course needs to taste great. Gravies, sauces, and dressings are areas where the More Flavor Family members will consume an inordinate amount of calories. Unlike those of us in the More Food Family, who are more concerned with volume, the More Flavor folk can't stand the thought of eating bland food— it just doesn't satisfy them. They need the "zing" of really tasty morsels and can easily lose control when they encounter something delicious. The More Flavor Family would prefer blue cheese dressing to low-fat Italian. Obviously, at 140 calories for two teaspoons of blue cheese, portion control is of the utmost importance if members of this family are to maintain a healthy weight.

FOOD FAMILIES MODIFICATION GUIDELINES

Before you create your weekly meal plan, decide what Food Family you're in and keep some guidelines in mind. If you're in the Food Is Fuel Family, you won't really need to make a lot of modifications to reduce your calories. General guidelines include replacing regular soda with water, eating more fresh fruits and vegetables rather than refined carbohydrates during the filler part of your meal, and avoiding high-sugar desserts, which will cause a feeling of sluggishness when the food is digested.

If you are in the More Food Family, your weekly meal plan may look quite different from your present weekly menu. You will be focusing on substituting leaner-fat, lower-carbohydrate, lower-calorie foods for the foods you currently eat. Instead of macaroni and cheese, try mashed cauliflower. Instead of a regular cheeseburger, try a lean hamburger without the bun. I also advocate using certain substitutes such as Splenda or diet soda or water to lower overall calories while maintaining or achieving higher food volume.

Eventually we will progress toward cleaning up our diets in terms of making healthier overall choices, such as organic and hormone-free foods. One thing I will not ask of you is to force yourself to reduce portion sizes dramatically. There is no need for that with this program. However, over time your portion sizes may naturally get smaller.

If you're in the More Flavor Family, your weekly meal plan may not be too different from what you're eating now. You may just need some small modifications to reach your goal of reducing your intake to reach your Personal Daily Fuel Goal.

Focus on portion control and substituting out the white poisons— sugar, salt, and flour—as well as starches, which contribute to belly fat. You should work on substituting foods that keep blood sugar levels stable, such as almonds and other nuts, lean meats and fish, berries, olive oil, eggs, and green leafy vegetables.

Whatever family you're in, if you focus on making good meals that are the same portion size yet are within your calorie range, you will naturally begin to eat more fruits and veggies. That's because when you have a caloric checkbook (which we discussed in Chapter 6), you've got a certain number of calories that you can spend every day on food. Make your goal the same as mine—to fit as much food as possible into your caloric budget. If you do that, you're naturally going to gravitate toward low-calorie options like fruits and vegetables.

By practicing Modification Not Starvation, you will find many different options, regardless of what family you're in. The key is that you stick with it, and I'll tell you why.

As I said before, I study weight-loss literature constantly to try to improve my knowledge base. I have reviewed many studies over the years that have compared the success of various weight loss programs. While it seems like groups on lower-carbohydrate plans seem to lose more weight than others in the short term, there are many variables that lead to long-term success. None of these variables even comes close to the importance of sticking with the program. Do the dieters stay on the program they begin, or do they stray? Researchers call this compliance. Greater compliance is very important because it has real-world value. You have to be able to stick with the particular program that you're on. That's why I recommend that you use Lose It Fast, Lose It Forever to create your own plan that fits your goals and lifestyle. Use mine as a blueprint or a guide.

Understand how I came up with it, then design your own so that you can maintain it permanently.

CREATING YOUR OWN WEEKLY FOOD PLAN

Now it is your turn to create your own weekly food plan. To make it easier, review your food journals from the past few weeks. You should notice and highlight certain normal, and maybe even abnormal, patterns of eating. For example, do you eat the same breakfast daily? Do you have weekly pizza with the family on Friday nights? These should all be taken into account as you come up with a weekly menu.

We need to be honest and include special considerations in our meal plan so that we don't experience the frustration of failure every week. If every Thursday you go out to a restaurant with your sister, you must write that into your meal plan. You're going to figure out in advance exactly what you can eat at the restaurant and incorporate it into your plan. Maybe you'll include a lighter lunch so you can spend your calorie budget at dinner.

Once we figure out our meal plan, including any special circumstances we may face, we are going to stick with it. That's because there is enough variety built into the plan that we can achieve our Forever Goals, but also there's enough variety in the plan that we should never feel like we're being deprived of anything.

The form below is available at www.PeteThomas.com, or you can create a chart like this in your LIF2 Success Journal. Remember to incorporate the Three Fs at every meal.

MY WEEKLY MEAL PLAN—BREAKFAST (LUNCH/DINNER)

	Fluid	Filler	Feast
Sunday			
Monday			
Tuesday			
Wednesday			
Thursday			
Friday			
Saturday			

Now that you have developed your weekly menu, you will need to go grocery shopping on a regular basis to stick to your plan.

SHOPPING FOR FOREVER

When I go grocery shopping, my focus is on Correct Calories, Cautious Carbs, so I am very cautious when it comes to the white poisons: sugar, flour, and salt. Whenever I have struggled with my weight I simply refer back to my list and start noticing the foods that I have been eating that are not on my list. Then I get back on track by going back to shopping only from my list. I practice two important principles that I want you to adopt. The first is that a modification or substitute for all of your favorite foods must be on your list. The second is this: *If it's not on the list, I must resist.*

Here is a sample of my personal shopping list. It takes time and experimentation to develop your own personal grocery list, but believe me, it is a core Forever Habit and essential for losing it forever. I constantly add foods to my personal grocery list when I find foods that fit within my criteria.

PETE'S GROCERY LIST

Description	Items
Meat, Poultry—and Seafood	
Breakfast	Turkey bacon—all-natural, uncured
	Canadian bacon
	Turkey maple breakfast sausage
Lunch/Snacks	Bologna (95% lean)
	Chicken wings (teriyaki lime)
	Turkey hot dogs
	Turkey pepperoni
	Ham (97% lean)
	Turkey breast (97% lean)
	Tuna packed in water
Dinner	*
Fish and Seafood	Shrimp, tilapia, whitefish, etc.
	Pork loin—boneless
	Ground beef (96% lean)
	Chicken breasts—boneless/skinless

Description	Items
	Chicken thighs—boneless/skinless
	Turkey sausage
	Extra-lean ground turkey
	Lean turkey burgers
	Steak—sirloin
Snacks	Cool Whip Free and Cool Whip Sugar-free
	Fat-free Reddi-wip (light blue cap, not red)
	Sugar-Free Popsicles
	No-Sugar-Added Fudgsicles
	Sugar-Free Jell-O
	Low-carb yogurt such as Carbmaster or Light & Fit
	Low-fat yogurt
	Pickles
	Laughing Cow Cheese (Light 3-pack)
	Strawberries
	Cherries
Drinks	Diet Rite
	Diet Orange Sunkist (bottles or 2-liter)
	Crystal Light
Condiments	Miracle Whip Light
Spices/Supplies	Pam cooking spray
	Reduced-sugar ketchup
	Mustard—yellow
	I Can't Believe It's Not Butter! spray
	Chile and corn salsa
	Tomato-less salsa
	Mrs. Dash
	Lawry's Seasoned Salt
Bread	Low-carb tortillas
	Light whole grain bread
Dairy	Laughing Cow Cheese (Light 3-pack)
	Egg Beaters / egg whites
Fruits and Vegetables	Cherries
	Strawberries
	Melons
	Lemons
	Spinach (canned)

	Lima beans (canned)
	Greens (canned)
	Frozen vegetables
Salad Items	Lettuce
	Bell peppers (red/yellow/green)
	Tomatoes—cherry or grape
	Onions
	Green onions
	Garlic
	Cucumbers
	Jalepeño peppers
	Banana pepper rings
	Carrots
	Mushrooms
	Sweet peas
	Raisins
	Dried cranberries
	Sunflower seeds
	Water chestnuts
	Red cabbage
	Pickles
	Olives—black and green
	Low-fat Italian dressing
	Miso Dijonnaise Dressing

If you don't find all the foods you want on my list, consult the list in the Fluid, Filler, and Feast section on page 117. As you find good alternatives to your regular groceries, come and tell the rest of us about it at www .PeteThomas.com.

WHICH LABEL TO BELIEVE?

Learning to grocery shop differently involves training yourself to think about nutrition in a new way, as well as reading labels in a new way. The first thing you need to do is compare the nutrition labels on the different brands. These are the labels on the back of the box or can. When you do this, be sure to keep an eye on the serving size and the calories.

I want you to pay attention to the back label, because sometimes the front label can be deceptive. When you read that something is fat-free or sugar-free, you need to remember that flavor has to come from some-where. So if it says it's fat-free, where does the flavor come from? It prob-ably comes from added sugar or salt, or both. If it says it's sugar-free, where does the flavor come from? It probably comes from added fat, salt, or some other flavoring. You really want to be careful about these two things, because fat-free and sugar-free do not mean calorie-free.

Shopping differently takes practice, just like eating differently takes practice. In the Challenges section at the end of this chapter, you will find my Grocery Store Scavenger Hunt, which I invented for my weight loss students. It's a fun way to practice grocery shopping the healthier way. Here are some things to consider as you shop for groceries:

- **Switch brands**—If you don't like the taste of one brand, try another brand or manufacturer, but don't go back to the old, calorie-rich version.
- **Ratchet it down**—Compare all the options in one food type and try the one with the lowest possible number of calories. Try light, fat-free, sugar-free, and so on.
- **Middle of the road**—Balance calories and taste; if you can't stand any of the low-calorie versions of a food, try one that is middle of the road (like the jam example I explained earlier—first low sugar, then no sugar).
- **Switch up items**—If there are no low-calorie versions of a food that you like, switch to a different type of food and leave the old one behind. For example, you may consider a switch from mayonnaise to mustard.

CREATE YOUR PERSONAL GROCERY LIST

Now you are finally ready to create your personal grocery list. You can get ready for this by completing the Grocery Store Scavenger Hunt from the Challenges section. Then use the suggested foods list to help fill in your own list. Revise your shopping list regularly as you experiment with dif-ferent foods and condiments. And remember the principle I mentioned: "If it's not on the list, I must resist."

Organize your list, using the following:

- Meat, poultry, fish, and seafood
- Vegetables
- Fruits and snacks
- Bread and dairy
- Condiments and spices

Also it may be easier to organize your list by breakfast, lunch, and dinner. Now that you know how to make a shopping list, go ahead and make your own using the principles you've learned. You can download blank shopping lists at www.PeteThomas.com.

YOU DID IT

Look at you. You've created a personalized weekly meal plan and a detailed grocery list. Take a minute to digest that accomplishment. You are well on your way to eating differently and losing it forever. Our goal is permanent change, not temporary restrictions, so pat yourself on the back.

So many diets tell you what and when to eat. But together we were able to create our own meal plan and timetable. We've fashioned a plan that we can make work under any circumstances. You are well on your way to significant, life-changing weight loss.

Congratulations!

KEY POINTS

- Lose It Fast, Lose It Forever offers the best of both worlds by incorporating the variety of a counting plan (in which you can eat anything you want as long as it is within caloric limits) and the discipline of a set plan (repeating our favorite nutritious foods over and over to keep us within our goals).
- Losing some weight is not our goal; learning to eat *correctly* for the *rest of our lives* is the real goal.

- The main purpose of figuring out how many times you're going to eat is so that you can maintain your energy level by maintaining even blood sugar levels.
- People fall into one of these Food Families based on their attitude toward food and eating habits: the Food Is Fuel Family, More Food Family, and More Flavor Family.

CHAPTER 8 CHALLENGES

Grocery Store Scavenger Hunt

Now for some fun. You need to go to the grocery store. Trust me, this will be enjoyable. Go through your local full-service grocery store and select a high-calorie food and a low-calorie food from the list below. All items must be of comparable serving sizes. Write down the brand, the serving size, and the calories. You can download this form from www .PeteThomas.com, or write down your answers in your food journal.

MEATS

Select the highest-calorie breakfast meat (example: bacon, brand X,
   2 slices, 80 calories)
Select the lowest-calorie breakfast meat (example: bacon, brand Y,
   2 slices, 40 calories)

SALAD DRESSING

Select the highest-calorie salad dressing
Select the lowest-calorie salad dressing

BREADS

Select the highest-calorie bread or wrap
Select the lowest-calorie bread or wrap

DRINKS (NONALCOHOLIC)

Select the highest-calorie drink
Select the lowest-calorie drink

SANDWICH SPREADS

Select the highest-calorie sandwich spread

Select the lowest-calorie sandwich spread of the same type

SNACKS

Select the highest-calorie yogurt

Select the lowest-calorie yogurt

CHEESE

Select the highest-calorie cheese

Select the lowest-calorie cheese

DESSERT FOODS

Select the highest-calorie cold dessert food

Select the lowest-calorie cold dessert food

Write Your Top 5 Daily Food Modification List

Once you've checked out your local grocery store for practical modifications, make a list of your Top 5 Modified Foods. These should be foods
that you eat frequently. Be as specific as possible with the old brands, the
new brands, and the calories per serving size.

"I dropped ten sizes after taking LIF2. I have a pair of shorts that I wore at Disney last year, and I get to go back this year, almost a year later, to redo some of our key pictures and I get to wear clothes that are ten sizes smaller . . . *so that's awesome."*

—CARMEN, LIF2 STUDENT

TIPS FOR ENTERTAINING, EATING OUT, AND ENJOYING THE HOLIDAYS

PEOPLE ASK ME, "DO YOU STILL EAT OUT?" OF COURSE I DO, LIKE everybody else. I do a lot of traveling and speaking, which means I don't always have the opportunity to prepare my own meals. Many people face this challenge, especially people who travel frequently for their jobs. Like I said in Chapter 6, a diet plan is only good if it works in the real world. So let me explain the principle of Modification Not Starvation as it relates to eating out.

EATING OUT WITHOUT PIGGING OUT

Let's say you went to Burger King, which is a nationwide chain. Now if you are saying to yourself, "I would never go to Burger King!" then you are a healthier eater than most. But the principle that I am about to apply here will help you no matter where you eat. A Whopper with cheese is 770 calories. If you modify the Whopper by replacing the bun with lettuce, you save 240 calories; if you replace the mayo with mustard, you save 160 calories; and if you replace the cheese with extra pickles and tomatoes, you save 90 calories. You can knock that Whopper with cheese all the way down from 770 calories to 280. By practicing Modification Not Starvation I can still enjoy my burger—and maintain my weight by saving calories along the way.

Now you may be thinking to yourself, "But I like the bun!" So I ask you—when was the last time you ordered a bun by itself? Or better yet, when was the last time you went to the pantry and ate a plain hamburger or hotdog bun with nothing on it? I am willing to bet your reply is "never." Most of us do not like a plain bun. We like a bun mixed with juice from the meat (otherwise known as grease), mayonnaise, mustard, pickle juice, and ketchup. But is the bun non-negotiable? If we can save some calories by taking certain things off and combining other things with it, we're going to be better off and we're still going to be able to enjoy the things that we really like in life. This is Modification Not Starvation in practice.

Whenever I travel to the West Coast, I make sure I stop at In-N-Out Burger, because they serve one of their burgers "protein style." Basically what they do is take the hamburger off the bun and wrap it in lettuce. That's almost perfect; if you can make another substitution and have them take off the mayo and put on mustard, you're saving even more calories. Then it's perfect.

Some of us are "dessert people," while others are into "salt" or "sweet and sour," and still others are "meat and potatoes" type folk. I'm a "meat and meat" kind of guy. If I can have two hamburgers, I'll trade in that baked potato with sour cream. The strength of this program is that it is adaptable to our real lives. That means we've got to decide what things we really want and what we can substitute, which is why we write things down and track our calories.

Here are a few more modifications for when you're eating outside of the home:

- Get rid of the bread or the bun.
- Substitute the mayo and/or cheese.

- Substitute any other sauces that are put on sandwiches, or ask for them without the sauce.
- Order your low-cal salad dressing and cheese on the side and use them sparingly.
- Trade your fries for fruit or salad or both.
- Look for the words "grilled," "baked," or "broiled" on the menu instead of "fried" (yes, you can learn to say no to fried chicken!).
- Ask for an egg white omelet instead of a traditional omelet, or even an Egg Beaters omelet.
- Select lower-calorie meats; for example, Canadian ham rather than regular ham, and turkey bacon rather than pork bacon.
- When it comes to good old American pizza, select thin crust rather than thick crust.
- You can also order half-and-half—for example, order the omelet with half eggs, half egg white.

If you can follow these suggestions when you're eating out, you won't veer off course from pursuing your Forever Habits.

TOP TIPS FOR EATING OUT

Here are my tips for eating out:

- Go online and plan your meal ahead of time from the restaurant's website.
- Budget your calories in advance if you know that you're going to a place where you can't get around calorie-dense foods. And then only eat foods that you can measure.
- Carry your calorie-counting book with you or have a smart phone app available whenever you go out.
- Drink a lot of water while you wait for your meal, so you won't feel as hungry when the food arrives.
- At the very beginning of the meal, take half of your meal and box it up. Caution—if it's a trigger food, this is dangerous, because you're going to be tempted to eat it on the way home. Trigger foods are specific foods that cause a person to overeat because he or she just

loses control. The most common trigger foods are sugar-fat combinations like ice cream and cookies, or fat-salt combinations such as French fries and potato chips. Some foods you don't want to box up and take home. If you order a trigger food, be careful not to take the extra food home with you. We may have the best intentions to take some of our meal and save it for the next day. But let's be honest, a trigger food probably will not make it through the night at home.

- If you're eating out with someone, each of you can order individual salads and then split the main course.
- Order your dressing on the side, and don't pour it on your salad. Better options would be to dip your salad in the dressing or dip your fork in the dressing and then stab your salad.
- Have your waiter take away items that you don't want to eat. For instance, if bread comes out and you know it's not good for you, have the waiter take it away. You can also ask the server beforehand not to bring out things you don't want.
- Have extra food quickly removed from the table. As you are finishing something and you know that you're almost full, tell the waiter to take it away.
- Redirect your group to a healthier restaurant, where you can better determine your calories. Trust me, you can do it!

TIPS FOR ENTERTAINING

Hosting or attending parties can be a minefield for dieters. So let me give you some tips for entertaining:

- After cooking up treats to serve guests, make up a care package of extra treats to send home with each guest so that you get rid of all the extra food from your house. Like everyone else, you want to poison your family and friends by overloading them with cakes and cookies— I understand that. But when the party is over, send it all home with your guests.
- The corollary to this is that if your guests bring treats with them, make sure the treats go home with them.

- When making or buying the food, mix in healthy dishes so there are options that fit into your own Forever Habits. Some examples are "protein style" lean hamburgers (without a bun or in a low-carb wrap), lower-calorie lasagna, and lean pork loin dishes (you can find this and other recipes on www.PeteThomas.com).
- Add up the calorie totals in your own recipe or dish. Then divide the dish into equal serving sizes, so that you know how many calories you are taking in.

Eating out or attending a party does not need to be the death of your Forever eating habits. Remember, Lose It Fast, Lose It Forever is not an elimination diet where you get rid of entire food groups. You can reasonably eat what you want within your calorie budget. Have fun on your way to losing those Forever Few!

TIPS FOR ATTENDING A PARTY

- Eat a big meal before attending the party, preferably with lots of fillers like vegetables or soup. If you're not hungry when you arrive, you'll be less tempted to binge on the fatty, sugary foods normally encountered at parties.
- Avoid fasting on the day of a party. Some people are tempted to save all their calories for the special event—we talked in Chapter 8 about why that's not a good idea. Eat your meals, but reduce the calories at those meals so that you have some calories left in your checkbook when you arrive at the sugar fest.
- Limit the alcoholic drinks you consume. Most people make the mistake of thinking all of their calories are coming from the food, but alcoholic drinks can pack a lot of calories. Switch to soda water or diet soda and save your calories for those special foods you want.
- Plan to stay on your plan. Don't "quit for the holidays." Remember, this is not a diet, this is a lifestyle. You can have some sweets, but stick to your daily calorie budget.
- Increase your exercise during holiday season. This will not only keep you looking good; it also will allow you to eat a few more calories at the parties.

- Wear something that fits you well and shows off your newly slimmed figure. Enjoying how great you look will help motivate you to keep the weight off.
- Keep moving around—talk to other guests, help serve, play games, dance—just don't sit in a corner and eat. For many people, boredom = snackdom.
- Use a smaller plate so you will have to stop piling food on.
- Learn to forgive yourself if you eat too much, and make some minor adjustments the next day.

YOU DON'T NEED TO CHEAT

Let me talk about cheat days for a minute, because many people think that cheating is the only way to approach going to a party or making it through the holidays. Many plans promote a high-calorie or cheat day, or what some have called a "fat day" as a way to fight the feeling of depriving yourself throughout the week. I am totally against this idea, for several reasons.

I remember one time I was on a diet for which they allowed you to have a cheat day on Saturday. Whenever I had a cheat day, I would drive over an hour to the nearest Uno Pizzeria and have my very own deep-dish, meat lover's, Chicago-style pizza. Not a slice—a whole pizza. All to myself. With a Diet Coke. It was so emotionally fulfilling that my cheat day would turn into an entire cheat weekend, and before long, it had turned into a cheat week. Pretty soon my diet died from all the cheating.

In addition, cheat days can destroy the gains you have achieved throughout the week. For example, let's say that you have cut back by 500 calories a day from Sunday through Friday for a total of 3000 calories. You are doing well and you are scheduled to lose about 1 pound that week because 3500 calories equals 1 pound. But on your cheat Saturday you consume an extra couple thousand calories. If you have not completely erased all of that week's weight loss, you're pretty close to it. Or look at it another way—in one day you have just wiped out four days of effort.

Last, the concept of a cheat day treats food as a reward. One of our Forever Habits is that we have come to understand that food is fuel. That's all it is. It is a need. We should reward ourselves with things that contribute to better health and help us to fulfill our purpose in life. These rewards can include massages, new shoes or clothes, a new hairstyle, great times with friends and family, trips and vacations, special nights out on the town, and so on. Food should never become the reward itself.

In case our discussion has not convinced you thus far, let me say one more thing about using food as a reward. We reward dogs with food. Consider that the next time you offer your child a food reward for a job well done.

There is a solution to a cheat day. If you want a particular item, you can simply budget for it that day. Do you have an uncontrollable craving for an oatmeal raisin cookie? Put it into your daily calorie budget and have it sometime during that same day. My goal is to minimize my crazy sugar cravings, but to be honest sometimes I do fit a cookie into my day. That's what is so amazing and wonderful about this plan. If you pay attention to your Daily Fuel Goal and you budget out your calories, eating what you want will never be "cheating." I want to illustrate further what I mean by telling you a little Christmas story.

CHRISTMAS CONFECTIONS

For many years, I would go to a good friend's house in Chicago for Christmas. His last name is Baker; the name was perfect for him because he made wonderful desserts. Everything he made was delicious, but the desserts were absolutely heavenly—and very high calorie. After I lost my weight, I knew that I would have to plan my calories correctly when I went to visit him.

I tried all different sorts of tricks and methods to make sure I could stay within my calories and still eat my friend's desserts. I would skip dinner the night before. I would skip breakfast and lunch the day of and wait to eat for dinner. I would skip lunch. I would try to completely resist the desserts. None of these things worked very well, and I always ended up overeating. Finally I said, "Okay, I'm going to have just a little bit of breakfast, just a little bit of lunch, and then at dinnertime I'm going to have what I really want." At dinner I would have very small portions of fluids and fillers and go straight for the desserts, because those were what I really wanted.

Now, was that the most nutritious way to eat that week? Of course not. But it worked for me for a few days during Christmas. The most important thing for me was to not go over my calories. I would pick and choose a little piece of every single dessert, and then I would go back for seconds on the desserts I really liked. The next day I would be so pleased. The Old Pete would have had a normal big breakfast, a normal big lunch, and then at dinnertime would have just stuffed himself on all the dinner foods, and then rolled around picking at all the desserts. And then rolled around all evening in the discomfort that came from overstuffing himself.

I tell you this story to illustrate that you need to develop a plan that works for you. We've got to experiment. And we need to learn how to plan in advance for a party. Think in advance about your night out, so none of those situations take you by surprise.

KEY POINTS

- A diet plan is only good if it works in the real world—for instance, eating out at restaurants.
- If you pay attention to your Daily Fuel Goal and you budget out your calories, eating what you want will never be "cheating."
- We've got to decide what foods we really need and what we can substitute, which is why we write things down and track our calories.
- If we're making or buying the food for a party, we need to mix in healthy dishes.

CHAPTER 9 CHALLENGES

New Challenges | Create an Eating-Out Tip List

Write down some of your own top tips for eating out, so that you can be in control of your eating when you go to a restaurant. Share this list with the other people in your life, as well as with your food teammates.

Create an Entertaining Tip List

Write down some of your modification ideas for entertaining or hosting parties. Celebrating your weight loss would be a great reason to throw a party! Introduce your friends to healthy food. Who knows, you might be saving their lives, too! Share your tip list with the rest of the LIF2 community at www.PeteThomas.com.

Create a Tip List for How to Attend a Party

Write down some of your ideas for attending a party without giving up your weight loss program. Help others do the same by posting your list on my website.

Ongoing Challenges | Touch a Teammate

Don't forget, after you achieve your first weight loss success or your first Forever Habit, go to www.PeteThomas.com and trumpet your achievement. We want to hear about it, and your story could inspire someone else.

"My doctor was pushing bariatric surgery very hard, but I knew that there was a better way to lose weight. I have been on every program in the world, it seems like. They all worked to some extent, but I had never been able to change my lifestyle. Eventually I always fell back. Until Lose It Fast, Lose It Forever. Pete's program just makes sense. First and most important, I had to realize that I was truly worth the time that it would take to exercise. In the first seven weeks I lost 49 pounds. I know that anyone can follow the principles that Pete teaches."

—MIKE, LIF2 STUDENT

CHAPTER

10

MULTIPLY YOUR MUSCLES

LEARNING TO REALLY EXERCISE AT *THE BIGGEST LOSER* RANCH WAS so incredibly hard I wondered if I would survive it. We worked out for four hours each and every day.

These were not easy workouts, where we did a little bit of walking and then rested. Everything we did was high intensity. We'd start with overhead dumbbell presses and move on to push-ups, squats, jumping jacks, lunges, biceps curls, then back to squats, lunges, push-ups, and running up and down hills. Everything we did was very, very intense. It was nothing but hard work.

We did two types of workouts on the ranch: resistance workouts and aerobic (or cardiovascular) workouts. I'm going to tell you about both of these types of workouts and why they are so effective. But first, I'm going to discuss some of the benefits of exercise in general, so you'll be motivated to "Multiply Your Muscles" in a way that helps you lose weight both fast and forever.

WHY EXERCISE?

We have two goals when it comes to exercise. The first is to be healthy. In other words, we want to develop a habit of exercise that's related to fitness. The more physically fit we are, the longer we will live and the better the quality of life we will have. That's because regular exercise is good for your heart and helps lower your risk for conditions like high blood pressure and diabetes.

The second goal of exercise is weight loss, in which our goal is straight-up fat loss. We want to exercise for weight loss so that we can lose fat on our bodies. Safe, lasting weight loss occurs as we create a caloric deficiency through balanced nutrition and exercise. Technically, we could reduce our calories so much through dieting alone that we lose weight. However, there are certain benefits that come from exercise that just don't come from dieting alone.

We will lose weight and keep it off much more efficiently if we combine good nutrition with learning to exercise properly. Exercise accelerates weight loss because it burns up the extra fuel you have stored in your body. In a nutshell, exercise speeds up your metabolism and causes your body to burn calories during and after the workout. Exercise will also help you look your best by toning your muscles and enabling you to get rid of that excess flab.

We are going to see two kinds of exercise in this guide: cardiovascular exercise, which concentrates on working the heart and lungs; and resistance training, which uses weight of some kind to build the other muscles of the body. My goal is to teach you how to combine cardio and resistance training to achieve maximum fat burning. Not only will exercising allow us to consume more calories a day, building muscle will actually help us burn calories long after our workouts have ended. Very simply, muscle burns more calories than fat, partly because it takes energy to repair your muscles after an intense workout.

Building muscle is even more important as we get older. As we age, our bodies require less fuel because the muscles in the body deteriorate or atrophy without regular use. As this happens, the need for fuel is also reduced, meaning you will require fewer calories. Muscles are the metabolic engine of the body, and resistance training increases and maintains that metabolic engine. As we maintain our muscles, we increase or maintain the number of calories we need to consume on a daily basis.

Exercise has even more benefits besides the two I've just mentioned. One is that it increases your endorphin and serotonin levels. These hormones are called "God's natural antidepressants." Exercise also relieves stress, increases energy, and improves your focus. Exercise can also be fun, which contributes to a better quality of life. So there are many reasons to exercise, if your doctor gives you permission to participate.

But the bottom line for us is that exercise allows you to accelerate your weight loss.

WEIGHT LOSS MATH

Let me give you some weight loss math. How do we lose weight through exercise? It's very simple. Remember I told you that 3500 calories equals 1 pound. If you're like me, you may not love math, but that is a very important equation for you to understand:

3500 calories = 1 pound

It follows, then, that if we burn 500 calories a day through exercise over the course of seven days, that's going to equal just about 1 pound lost per week.

Burn 500 calories per day × 7 days = 1 pound per week of weight loss

But the real question is how do we accomplish this? How can we burn 3500 extra calories in a week?

F.I.T.T.—PETE'S SPECIAL ACRONYM

After I came back from *The Biggest Loser* Ranch, I was looking for some simple way to quantify and describe what we did on the show. So I pulled a whole bunch of variables together: the types of exercises, how often we did them, how hard we worked out, and several others. I called it by some fancy name. I was so proud of myself! I even developed an acronym for it that I have since forgotten.

Then I discovered something called F.I.T.T. It's actually a very common principle that's taught to a lot of trainers, although many trainers neither teach it to their clients nor go into enough depth to really help someone long-term. So allow me. F.I.T.T. stands for:

Frequency
Intensity
Time
Type

Frequency

How many days a week are you going to work out? Like I said in Chapter 1, you need to take some time for yourself on a regular basis. How many days a week can you invest in some solid exercise time? On *The Biggest Loser* Ranch, we worked out for six days a week. On our "rest day," Jillian made us do things like climb a mountain. Some rest day! I'll tell you that story in Chapter 13.

You, too, will have an active rest day. On an active rest day you take the kids to a museum or the zoo, or you may go shopping. You're walking around and being active, although you are not elevating your heart rate too much.

If you work out six days a week—which is the frequency I'm suggesting to really see results—then you will need to take an off day. You're going to start with some pretty intense cardiovascular exercise, so you're giving the body a chance to recover on your off day.

You may be asking yourself, "Why did you guys work out so very hard on *The Biggest Loser*?" The answer is simple—we had ambitious goals. Our goal was to lose 1 pound a day or more. You also have a goal, but yours is to Lose It Forever by developing Forever Habits. Regular exercise is one of those Forever Habits.

I know from having taught this method for several years now that, at this point, some of you are getting nervous. You're asking, "Do I personally have to work out that hard and that long each day?" Well, it all depends on your weight loss goals. How much weight do you want to lose? How quickly do you want to lose it? Whether you have 15 pounds or 150 pounds to lose, applying the F.I.T.T. principle to your daily life will cause you to lose the weight at the pace you determine. As I said, I would like you to work out six days a week, even if you are in Step 4: Your Purpose, because you will really see great results at that frequency. In Step 1: Your Power, I asked you to start by working out twice in a week if you had not been exercising at all. I would like you to work up to six days a week over the next few weeks. If you need help with that, I have provided several different workouts in Chapter 13 that you can refer to.

Intensity

Next is the "I" in F.I.T.T., which stands for Intensity. By intensity I do not mean impact. I am talking about how hard you are working out based on your heart rate. We need to figure out how hard we should be working out. Over the past few years I have observed an unproductive focus on "calorie burn" in weight loss circles. Some of this has even been fueled by products that were featured on my favorite TV show. Allow me to correct your focus. If you work out at the correct intensity, your "calorie burn" will take care of itself. We need to focus on heart rate!

There are two different formulas I use for determining this. One formula comes from famous fitness author Dr. Phil Maffetone; I will explain this in Chapter 14 when we discuss running. For now, I'm going to stick with the central formula I used on *The Biggest Loser*. When it comes to intensity, I make sure that each one of my workouts averages around 85 percent of my maximum heart rate.

You know you're having a good workout if your heart rate stays around 85 percent of maximum. That's why it's very important for us to know exactly what our heart rate is throughout our workouts, which is why I asked you to purchase a good heart rate monitor back at the beginning of the book.

Some of you have never heard these terms before. Don't worry; it's pretty easy to understand. First, you need to figure out your maximum heart rate. That formula can be found on my website, www.PeteThomas .com. Or you can simply figure it out now.

For women, your maximum heart rate is 220 minus your age. You are going to work out within your aerobic range, which is 75 to 85 percent of your maximum heart rate. You're going to get the most benefit if your workout is at 85 percent of maximum and above. For men, your maximum heart rate is 226 minus your age. Your aerobic range will be 75 to 85 percent of your maximum heart rate, with emphasis on staying at the upper end of that range. Go ahead and write down your maximum heart rate, along with your aerobic range. It should look like this:

My maximum heart rate _____

My aerobic range _____

Keep in mind that maximum heart rate doesn't mean that you can never go above that number. You are not going to fall over dead if you suddenly hit this number. That number is more of a guideline than a rule. Knowing your maximum heart rate is going to help you have an effective workout.

While I'm talking about intensity, let me mention that there are two types of workouts. One is the fun kind. Playing catch in the backyard, golfing, and bowling would be examples of fun workouts. These are actually closer to what we would call activities rather than workouts. They get us moving around a little bit, and they're great for rest days, but they are relatively ineffective when it comes to weight loss.

The second kind of workout is an actual workout. Real workouts may not be fun, but they are absolutely effective in weight loss. The discussion in this chapter deals with the types of workouts that are rigorous. These are the kind during which we cannot read a magazine or talk on the phone. We need to elevate our heart rate and get a good sweat going—that's a real workout.

Time

The next initial in our F.I.T.T. principle stands for Time. Time is how many minutes a day and per session we should work out—which, again, depends on our goals. This program can work for anyone, whether you need to lose 20 for your daughter's wedding, or 120 to get rid of those obesity-related conditions.

I know that not everyone reading this book is out to Lose It Fast; I also know that not everyone reading this book needs to lose a massive amount of weight like I did. In short, we don't all need to exercise for the same amount of time, at the same intensity, and with the same variety of exercises. So when people ask me to give them recommendations for how much they should exercise, I say, "That depends on your goals and how much time you can dedicate toward those goals."

The government has some very basic recommendations for daily exercise. The Centers for Disease Control (CDC) lays out their most basic guidelines by recommending two hours and thirty minutes of exercise every week plus two additional days of resistance training a week.

I have found that this recommendation of approximately a half hour a day of exercise—which is fairly easy to schedule for most people—is a good starting point for maintaining your weight. It's better than sitting on the couch but won't lead to any real weight loss. That is a good maintenance workout—easy to fit in the schedule and possibly quite enjoyable, but that's about it for benefits.

The government takes it a little bit further by providing instructions for "even greater" health benefits. These guidelines include five hours of exercise every week plus two additional days of resistance training a week.

This last recommendation—five hours a week plus additional resistance training—comes closer to what I recommend, but it still may not provide you with much weight loss if you don't exercise intensely using the correct type of workouts.

If you want to lose weight fast or forever, you'll need to bump up your workouts to an hour a day minimum. On my plan you perform your ABC Circuits on Monday, Tuesday, Thursday, and Friday, with Wednesday and Saturday being cardio days. Sundays will be your (active) rest days. We'll talk about this plan in more detail in Chapter 13.

Even the government notes that "more time equals more health benefits." Remember, to Lose It Forever you will have to honestly assess your goals and dedicate time to reaching those goals. Applying the F.I.T.T. formula will go a long way in helping you to do just that.

Results show—and my own experience demonstrates—that sixty to ninety minutes a day, five to six days a week, is going to yield 1 to 2 pounds of weight lost a week. I call this "average weight loss."

If you have more ambitious goals and work out 150 minutes a day—that's two and a half hours—six days a week, you're going to lose right around 1 percent of your body weight a week. I call this "excellent weight loss." If you work out that much a day, you will approach *Biggest Loser* "home" results. When the contestants on *The Biggest Loser* are voted off and sent home, those who work out intensely two and a half hours a day lose about 1 percent of their body weight a week. For someone weighing 350 pounds, that equals 3½ pounds of weight loss a week, or 91 pounds in six months. I know that two and a half hours of exercise sounds like a lot, but I broke it up by doing one sixty-minute session in the morning and another ninety-minute session after work at night.

Sometimes your immediate weight loss is going to be more dramatic than what you would expect. Then the pace will level off as your body settles in. Even after that, though, you can still see excellent weight loss results based on your desire to follow these guidelines.

Now if your goals and your schedule will allow you to work out for 240 minutes—four hours—a day, six days a week, you're going to achieve "superior weight loss." This superior weight loss is going to be similar to *Biggest Loser* Ranch results. While I was at the ranch, we worked out very intensely at 85 percent of our maximum heart rate and above for four hours, six days a week. We lost, on average, 2 to 3 percent of our body weight a week. I'll show you how to convert these numbers to a formula in a minute.

Things have changed a little bit on *The Biggest Loser* regarding time and intensity. A few seasons ago, they decided to exchange some intensity for time. In other words, the contestants worked out with lower intensity but added more time. This has yielded good results, but I prefer to spend less time exercising, so I am sticking with the higher intensity and lower time. In other words, I recommend that you work out as hard as possible for as long as possible and then get out of the gym and enjoy life.

HOW LONG WILL THIS TAKE ME?

Our goal is to make changes in our habits that lead to losing those extra pounds, then repeating those actions over and over until we've lost that Forever Five and even more. I probably shouldn't even include the following formula because Forever Habits are not something we drop when we've reached our goal weight. But for those who want to have some idea when they will complete their long-term goal, I will include it. If you don't care so much about when you will finish, skip this section and go on to the next section.

This formula enables you to calculate how many pounds you can lose in a year, based upon the number of hours a day that you're willing to work out.

WEIGHT LOSS TIMELINE

How Time Much Time Per Day Should I Work Out?			
30 minutes a day, 5 to 6 days a week	=	maintain current weight	
60 to 90 minutes a day, 5 to 6 days a week	=	average weight loss	= 1 to 2 pounds a week
150 minutes a day, 6 days a week	=	excellent weight loss (*Biggest Loser* home results)	= 1% a week (your weight x .01 = pounds lost)
240 minutes a day, 6 days a week	=	superior weight loss (*Biggest Loser* Ranch results)	= 2% to 3% a week (your weight x .025 = pounds lost)

Say your starting weight is 350, and you are willing to exercise 150 minutes, five to six days a week. Here is how much you will lose per week and per year assuming you have also adjusted your nutritional intake to support your exercise efforts.

We will take your initial weight and move the decimal point two places to the left, which leaves us with 3.5. With 150 minutes of exercise per week, your estimated weekly weight loss would be 3½ pounds a week. How much could you lose in a year? Multiply the 3.5 by 52 weeks, and that equals 182 pounds in one year, very similar to what I lost in my first year of weight loss. Of course, this formula only works up until you reach your goal weight; then you would make new maintenance goals and work out in a manner more appropriate for Your Purpose.

SHORTER OR LONGER WORKOUTS?

Another question that people ask me is this: What's best for working out, shorter workouts or longer workouts? Are two thirty-minute workouts better than one sixty-minute session? What I've discovered is that sixty minutes of continuous exercise is much, much better than two thirty-minute workouts a day.

When we exercise, our bodies begin to burn through our various energy stores. Research suggests that for the first thirty to forty-five minutes of a workout, energy is mainly provided by the glycogen present in our muscle and liver cells. Glycogen is the "storage" form of glucose, which is the form of sugar that our food is broken down into by our digestive system. After about forty-five minutes, the body begins to pull from our fat stores, converting the fatty acids to energy. The liver works to actually pull the fat out of our tissue and converts it to energy. So longer workouts will actually help you burn more fat than shorter workouts. In my experience, the absolute best workouts I've ever had for fat loss and weight loss are between ninety minutes and two hours. That seems to be optimal for amazing results.

If your schedule doesn't give you this much focused time, and you have to work out twice a day for thirty minutes, the key for you will be very, very intense workouts. If you can rearrange your schedule and turn those two sessions into one sixty-minute workout, you're going to see better results. But in the end, getting some workouts in is better than getting no workouts in at all.

PUTTING "ME TIME" ON YOUR SCHEDULE

Students ask me, "When is the best time to exercise? Should I exercise first thing in the morning or late at night?" That really depends. Some studies have shown that people who work out in the afternoon are able to put in harder workouts than those that choose the morning. But the fact of the matter is, there is one best time to work out—and that's when you can fit it in consistently. This program is designed around you and your schedule, so the best time for you to work out is when you can fit it all in. The point is for you to develop the Forever Habit of regular exercise, so that this new lifestyle stops feeling like a "diet."

Type

The last "T" in our F.I.T.T. principle is Type. What type of exercise should I be doing to reach my goals? That decision is very important. The next chapter deals with cardiovascular exercise, which is a great place to start if you're not already exercising. I'll cover resistance and weight training exercise in Chapter 12. When we begin to create our own Perfect Personalized Forever Workout Plan (Chapter 13), we will also want to consider in what order we do our cardiovascular or resistance training, as well as which body parts to work out on certain days. This is all part of deciding what type of exercise is right for our goals and lifestyle.

Let me say right here that, as with any diet or exercise program, you should see your doctor before you begin any workout program. Get his or her permission to participate in an exercise program.

KEY POINTS

- Safe, lasting weight loss occurs as we create a caloric deficiency through balanced nutrition and exercise.
- How fast you lose your weight depends on the F.I.T.T. principle. F.I.T.T. stands for:
  - Frequency
  - Intensity
  - Time
  - Type
- As with any diet or exercise program, you should see your doctor before you begin this workout program.

CHAPTER 10 CHALLENGES

New Challenges | Journal About Beginning to Exercise

Continue to write in your LIF2 Success Journal—only now let's start writing about exercising. Now that we know that 3500 calories burned equals 1 pound shed, answer the following questions:

- How frequently am I willing to exercise?
- How long am I willing to exercise?
- What type of exercise will I engage in? (You will have a better answer to this question after reading the next few chapters.)

Create a Weight Loss Timeline Using the Formula in This Chapter

If you want an estimate of how long it's going to take to reach your goal based on how much time you're willing to put in at the gym, calculate a rough timeline of when you'll reach your goal. Remember, this is only an estimate, and it is based on many different factors. My hope is that it will inspire you to stick with the Forever Habits you're forming and motivate you to spend that time exercising!

"Pete was able to cut through all the diet noise to provide real-life answers to questions so many of us have regarding food and exercise. With his help, I lost 35 pounds in the ten-week course, and 50 pounds over a four-month period. I've dropped my waist size from 44 to 36, my resting pulse rate from 68 to 52, my cholesterol from 257 to a 168, and my triglycerides from 352 to 191. Dropping from 280 pounds to 230 pounds has made a huge impact in the quality of my life. I have much more energy, and common tasks that were difficult or impossible are now far easier."

—GEORGE, LIF2 STUDENT

CHAPTER

11

KICK-START WITH CARDIO

AEROBIC EXERCISE PRIMARILY WORKS THE CARDIOVASCULAR SYSTEM, the heart, and lungs. We will be using the largest muscles in the body— the leg muscles—to work the heart and lungs and pull the fat out of the rest of the body. We will be covering two major types of cardiovascular exercise—steady state and interval training. First we'll talk about steady state.

STEADY STATE

Steady state cardio exercise is also known as Long Slow Distances (LSD), because some reasonably steady intensity is held for an extended period of time. Say, for instance, you run for twenty to sixty minutes at a heart rate of between 140 and 150 beats per minute in your aerobic range. That's what we mean by steady state—your heart is holding steady right around 140 or 150 beats per minute for an extended period of time.

Steady State Pros and Cons

Steady state cardio has both pros and cons. Here are some of the pros:

- It is great for beginners.
- It can be done daily, and even multiple times a day.
- When performed at the correct intensity, it can burn a great deal of calories during the workout session.
- It stimulates the release of endorphins, which are natural mood enhancers.
- As steady state becomes a part of a regular exercise regimen, it can help you stick to your diet. There are many reasons for this, including the fact that as you become more disciplined with exercise and start to feel better about your health, you will become more disciplined in your diet.

Steady state also has some drawbacks:

- It can be boring. To combat boredom, use a music player to break the monotony. I was so desperate on *The Biggest Loser* Ranch that I listened to the music other contestants had brought in when I got sick of my own. I remember jamming to a song by Hank Williams Jr. that said, "If the South woulda won we woulda had it made." That may have been an odd song for me to sing while working out, but I listened to just about anything to mask the sound of fat bodies sloshing around!
- An excess of endurance training can lead to muscle loss, as well as decreased power and strength—we will avoid this by combining resistance training with our cardio.
- Cardio can lead to overuse injuries if the exercise is not varied. You really need to do different types of cardiovascular exercise, like running, biking, elliptical, arc trainer, and swimming, to keep overuse injuries to a minimum.
- Small amounts of steady state are not very efficient for weight loss; if

you're going to do just thirty minutes a day of this type of exercise, you're not going to maximize your benefits.

HIGH-INTENSITY INTERVAL TRAINING

The other type of cardiovascular exercise is called interval training, or H.I.I.T. (high-intensity interval training), as it is known in some circles. This type of exercise combines a period of high-intensity effort with periods of lower intensity effort. And by "lower intensity" I don't mean you stop; you simply slow down.

A sample workout might start with a five-minute warm-up. That would be followed by thirty seconds of all-out effort, followed by four minutes and thirty seconds of slower effort within your aerobic range. Then back to thirty seconds of all-out effort, followed by four minutes and thirty seconds within your aerobic range. You will repeat this high-intensity/low-intensity pattern eight to ten times (fifty minutes) and then end with a five-minute cooldown.

You can do this H.I.I.T. routine on a bike or on a treadmill, or you could even do it walking or running outside. Let's say you've decided to use a treadmill. You are going to walk on a flat surface for four minutes and thirty seconds, and then you are going to raise the incline to a level 10 or 12 and you are going to walk uphill as fast as you possibly can for 30 seconds. Then, instead of stopping altogether, you are going to put the incline back down to a level grade and walk for four minutes and thirty seconds, after which you are again going to raise the incline to 10 or 12 and walk for another thirty seconds. You can find a number of specific H.I.I.T. cardio routines later in this chapter.

H.I.I.T. Pros and Cons

H.I.I.T. has advantages and disadvantages, just like steady state does. Here are some of the pros:

- This type of workout improves the body's ability to use fat as fuel.
- It is very, very efficient, because it yields a much greater calorie burn even during shorter workouts.

- It is never boring—you only have to stay focused for short periods of time.

But high-intensity interval training has some negatives as well:

- It can be difficult for beginners without proper training and guidance.
- For certain types of H.I.I.T. exercises you may have to schedule extra recovery time. In other words, you may be unlikely to have a hard interval run late one evening followed by another one the next morning.
- There is a higher potential for injury if you do the same type of exercise over and over again.

On *The Biggest Loser* Ranch we did high-intensity interval training every day of the week, but we did it using a variety of different exercises. One day we would be walking uphill on the treadmill or outdoors, the next day we would do intervals by riding a spin bike, and the next day we would walk on a stepper at varying speeds, followed by intervals on the elliptical, and then on the recumbent bike. Regardless of what you have heard, you can do intervals every day, as long as you vary the type of workout being performed.

The other great benefit of doing interval workouts, especially when you do them in the correct fashion, is something called EPOC. EPOC stands for excess post-exercise oxygen consumption. These are the calories burned after the exercise is finished. A great study done many years ago demonstrated that calories are burned up to thirty-six hours after certain types of interval workouts.

EXAMPLES OF CARDIO EXERCISE

Here are some examples of cardiovascular exercise. Many of them, like the exercises below, require no special equipment at all. They're basically calisthenics. I've explained the ones you may not be familiar with. You can try:

- Jogging
- Sprinting

- Squat hops (start with feet shoulder-width apart, arms at your side; do a regular squat with your back straight; from the squat, jump up as explosively as you can while reaching for the ceiling; when you land, lower your body back into the squat position)
- Jumping jacks
- Mountain climbers (start by getting on your hands and feet in a prone position like you're about to do a push-up; keeping your body parallel to the ground, alternate jumping your knees toward your chest)
- Squat thrusts (from a standing position, drop to a squat with hands on the floor in front of feet; kick feet back into a push-up position, then pull them quickly back up to a squat, then stand back up)
- Burpees (these are really squat thrusts with a jump added in; from a standing position, jump as high as possible; land on feet and place hands on the ground in front of you feet; kick you feet back into a push-up position and jump back up again to a standing position as fast as possible)
- Butt kicks
- High knees
- Jumping rope

Or you can get on a machine such as:

- A rowing machine
- A stair-climber (StairMaster)
- A treadmill
- A recumbent, upright, or spin bike
- An elliptical machine
- An arc trainer (a machine similar to an elliptical that combines elements of a climber, hiker, and skier)

Or you can go outside and walk or run up and down stadium stairs, jump rope, swim, ride your bicycle, or go for a hike.

I will provide examples of how to turn any of these exercises into an interval workout later in the chapter, as well as some sample workouts for you to start on. But first I want to cover a few important matters.

EATING FOR YOUR WORKOUT

I'm often asked, "Pete, should I eat before or after my workout?" It depends on how you feel. Let me give an example.

Every morning on *The Biggest Loser* Ranch, Dr. Jeff would go downstairs and get something to eat before he worked out. On his way down to the kitchen, he would knock on my door to wake me up. I would go to the bathroom and get dressed while he was eating. Then we would go to the gym together. I was able to put in a very good intense hour of working out without eating. Dr. Jeff needed some food in his stomach to be able to work out effectively. The important thing here is the quality of your workout and making sure that you have enough energy (i.e., food or fuel) to push through a complete workout. You need to feel good during the workout, neither light-headed and hungry nor too full with food sloshing around in your stomach. You need to experiment with this to get it right and see how you feel before your particular workouts.

The most common recommendations suggest that you consume approximately 200 to 400 calories two to three hours before the workout. Obviously this can be problematic if you have scheduled an early morning workout. Many times, dinner from the night before will hold you over until your workout is complete and it's time for breakfast. While most common recommendations advise a high-carbohydrate meal before exercise, I feel that this can be counterproductive to your Forever Habits. Many times I notice people consuming a high-sugar energy bar or something similar, using the excuse that they are going to "burn it off." I prefer a small meal such as a chicken breast salad with water, or a combo snack of almonds and a fruit (such as an apple) and water. Again, the real key is personal experimentation with the goal of powering through the workout.

I'm also asked, "Do I need to eat right after working out?" Many programs tell you to eat right after you work out. I do not necessarily agree with this advice and do not personally follow it. A lot of us have extra energy stored up (as fat), and a lot of the things we read and hear about are not really directed to people who need to lose a lot of weight. The advice to eat after a workout is mainly directed to athletes—people who have worked out incredibly hard and depleted themselves of a certain amount of energy. Athletes need to go out and refuel their bodies during an optimal time period, which is within the first hour after a workout.

If we are seriously trying to lose weight, we really need to consider whether or not this refueling is necessary. We definitely do not need to load ourselves back up with carbohydrates, because we want to avoid an unnecessary insulin increase, which may offset some of the other hormones released during exercise. If you do need to refuel, have a balanced meal, or, as a snack, eat lean protein like a tuna salad with a low-calorie dressing. Always be conscious of Correct Calories, Cautious Carbs, and have a fluid, a filler, and a feast. Remember, we don't want to cancel out the calories we just burned off during the workout we just put in.

EVEN WHALES HAVE ABS

One of my biggest pet peeves is when I am asked by people who are obese, "What type of exercise will trim down my stomach so I can see my abs?" or when someone says, "I am taking an abs class!" It bugs me to no end to go to the gym and see someone 50 pounds overweight wasting time doing crunches or sit-ups in an abs class. Do not take an abs-focused class or watch a video focused on your abs alone until your goal weight is within sight. Why? Because it's such a waste of time to focus on just one muscle group when no one will ever see it. Think about it—have you ever seen an obese person with really great abs? Look at my before picture—I had abs under there. No one ever saw it because I was as big as a whale.

Typically men will not see their abs until they're down to between 8 and 12 percent body fat and women between 12 and 15 percent body fat. So why focus on those muscles in advance of even being able to see them? My advice is to wait to take abs or sit-up classes until your goal is within sight. Your abs will be more visible once you lose the extra weight.

Now here's the one caveat to that: *Core exercises are a must,* and they are a part of this program. Exercises like the plank are a must. We want to work our core because we want to develop stability, so we want to work those muscles that support the back and the pelvis. This includes abs, but a focused abs class is literally a waste of time. You've only got so much time in the gym, so why spend thirty minutes of it in an abs class?

THE "P-WORD"

One of the most common questions I am asked is, "Will there be pain during my weight loss journey?" The truth of the matter is, yes, absolutely, there will be pain during your weight loss journey.

You may experience at least two different types of pain, just as I did on *The Biggest Loser*. Right up front, Jillian told me that I would experience both joint pain and muscle pain while I was on the ranch. The joint pain comes from your body having to adjust to the new stresses you're putting on it. So you're going to experience back pain, knee pain, and ankle pain. You will also experience muscle pain because you're working the muscles intensely. I was a little skeptical about what Jillian told me, but sure enough, I experienced joint pain from the start. She also predicted that within three weeks the joint pain would go away—and thank God it did.

Now here's the thing: Those three weeks on the ranch are equivalent to about three months in the real world. That's because we worked out more in the average week than most people work out in a month. But just like she said would happen, our large bodies got accustomed to all the extra stress we were putting on them and the joint pain went away.

I wish I could say the same thing about the muscle pain. But no, we pretty much had different muscle pain every single day. Different muscles were sore continuously because we were working those muscles like you wouldn't believe. Regular muscle soreness is a signal of the muscles breaking down and healing as a result of resistance exercise. We'll talk about that more in the next chapter. But the fact of the matter was that we always had some muscle pain.

When it comes to you and your weight loss journey, you've got to determine if you're experiencing joint pain or muscle pain, or whether you're suffering from an actual injury. If you're suffering from an injury, of course you need to go to the doctor and get that checked out.

You need to ask yourself a question about pain before you even begin: What will I do when I experience pain? I believe there are only a couple of ways to deal with it. You've got to:

- work through it
- work around it, or
- wrap it up

These are really your only options when it comes to pain that is not related to an injury. You'll have to work through it, work around it, or wrap it up.

During my time on *The Biggest Loser*, I used all types of things to help me endure the pain. I had several sizes of knee braces, heating pads, pain-killers, and medications like Preparation H for certain body parts that would get bothered in spin class. Throughout this process I learned one thing—I could work through it, work around it, or wrap it up and keep working.

The most amazing and helpful thing I discovered was that I was in pain not because I was working out, but because I was overweight. I finally figured that out because the more I worked out, the fewer braces I needed for my joints. I went from wearing a supersize brace on my knees (which now fits my thigh), to needing smaller and smaller braces, to not wearing any brace at all. The truth is, it was all that extra weight on my knees that was causing the problems, not the exercise itself.

TO GYM OR NOT TO GYM?

Should you work out at home or should you get a gym membership? There are pros and cons to each. The great advantage to working out at home is that it's convenient. As long as you can avoid any distractions, such as the kids or meal preparation or having to get work done, exercising at home can be very effective.

On the other hand, the great thing about working out at a gym is the abundance of equipment. In addition, whenever you're in an environment where everyone is working out, it typically causes you to work out just a little bit harder. The downside to a gym membership used to be the cost. But with some nationwide chains starting as low as $10 month (prices may vary), the benefits far outweigh the cost. Search around your local area to find a gym within your budget range. Remember that

YMCAs and schools often have great gyms that can be available to the public.

Do you need a trainer? In my personal opinion it's so easy to get a poorly trained or inexperienced trainer that it's not usually worth the expense. However, there are one or two specific times when a trainer can be absolutely vital to your success. You might want a trainer at the beginning of your weight loss efforts because she is going to show you how to properly do every exercise and how to safely work the equipment. Then at Step 3: Your Pursuit, it's going to be really helpful to have a trainer to help you shed those last few pesky pounds. But the truth is, while a trainer can be a vital part of your weight loss journey, we can lose weight with or without one—it all depends on how hard we are willing to work.

DRINKING ENOUGH WATER—IS THIS THE MAGIC WEIGHT LOSS ELIXIR?

You will need to keep yourself hydrated while you're working out. On the ranch, we drank approximately 16 ounces of water every fifteen minutes when we were working out. Water was a constant companion on the ranch. The common rule of thumb is to drink one half of your body weight in ounces a day. That means if you weigh 150 pounds, you need to consume 75 ounces of water a day. In general 100 ounces for men and 75 ounces for women should work, and that amount can be increased to a gallon a day when pushing through really hard stretches of exercise.

The importance of water cannot be understated. You can do without food and certain nutrients, but you cannot live without water. In some cases hunger is actually confused with dehydration. Many of us walk around in a constant state of dehydration. A glass here or there simply will not do the job. Dehydration can cause tiredness, muscle cramps, kidney problems, and many other conditions. Water boosts our energy, aids in metabolism, helps our organs absorb nutrients, and flushes out toxins and waste products from the body. Some health experts recommend drinking eight large glasses of water a day. If that's more than you drink now, then start with that. But not everybody is the same size, nor are we all involved in the same amount of activity during the day. Make a conscious effort to track your water consumption until drinking enough water becomes second nature.

WARM-UPS

We always want to warm up before we work out. The only time anyone in my season of *The Biggest Loser* ever got injured from working out was when a fellow contestant strained his leg muscles when we were rushing to film a *TV Guide* spot and didn't have a proper warm-up. So never skip your warm-up because you're in a hurry. The minimal time you should warm up for is at least five minutes of cardio followed by some simple dynamic stretches. Dynamic stretches, which are stretches that use continuous movement instead of holding a static end-point, help increase your range of motion and prep the muscles for action. You should look to actually break a sweat during your warm-up. Those who take my two-hour boot camp warm up for the first fifteen minutes with a variety of stretches.

PETE'S WARM-UP STRETCHES

Light Jogging

1. 75 percent max heart rate

Side Shuffles

1. Bend slightly at the knees and hips as you walk sideways, keeping your weight on the balls of your feet.
2. Walk one direction and then back, keeping the hips and knees level, without bouncing up and down.

Carioca with Twists

1. These are basically "grapevine" steps with a torso twist.
2. Step to the left with your left leg and immediately bring your right leg over and in front of the left leg and place it on the other side of the left leg.

3. While moving your right foot, twist your torso in opposition to the move of the leg so that your left shoulder ends up forward and facing to the right.
4. Bring your left leg up and over so that you are standing parallel again, twisting the torso in the opposite direction it just moved so that your right shoulder is forward.
5. Put your right leg on the other side of the left leg again, only go behind the foot this time, again twisting the torso in opposition.
6. Continue to repeat this alternating pattern, then switch directions.

High Knee Skips

1. Stand in place with feet hip-width apart.
2. Lift one knee up toward the chest and quickly place the foot back on the ground.
3. Repeat with the other knee.
4. Keep a fast pace with minimal ground contact time.

Butt Kicks

Jog while lifting the heels toward the butt with every step.

Knee Hug Walk

1. While walking forward, bring your left knee to the chest and pull the knee into the chest.
2. Repeat with your right knee.

That is just the preparation for the actual workout!

COOLDOWN STRETCHING

Let me be honest. I actually hate stretching because I want to maximize my exercise time. But stretching is very, very important, as it helps minimize soreness and speeds recovery. We will want to do the following seven basic static stretches for thirty seconds each whenever we exercise so that we are less likely to strain or pull a muscle. I usually do these at the end of my workouts.

Half Neck Rolls to the Front and Back

1. From the start position, very gently tip your head to the left. Pay attention to how your neck feels during this movement—if it is painful or your neck doesn't feel right, stop immediately.
2. Gently roll your head back into an extended position, with eyes facing the ceiling. This stretches and strengthens the muscles on the back of the neck.
3. With your head back, very gently roll your head to your right. If this is painful or your neck doesn't feel right, stop immediately.
4. Finish the stretch by rolling your head down again to the start position—head straight, eyes forward.

Standing Quad Stretch

1. Stand with a shoulder-width stance and hang on to an object or wall for support.
2. Bring one foot up behind you and grab the foot with your hand.
3. Pull your foot up toward your buttocks until you feel a stretch on the front of your thigh. Straighten your hip by moving the knee backward.
4. Hold and repeat on the other side.

Butterfly (inner thighs, groin, hips, lower back)

1. Sit up tall with the bottoms of your feet pressed together and your knees dropped to the sides as far as they will comfortably go.
2. Pull your abdominals gently inward and lean forward from the hips.
3. Grasp your feet with your hands and carefully pull yourself a little bit farther forward. You should feel the stretch spread throughout your inner thighs, the outermost part of your hips, and lower back.
4. Increase the stretch by carefully pressing your thighs toward the floor.

Hamstring/Back Stretch

1. Sit in an upright position. Tuck one foot near the groin with the opposite leg straight out.
2. Bending from the hips and leading with the chest, reach down until you feel a stretch in the back of the thigh.
3. Hold and repeat with the other leg.

4. Remember to keep the lower back straight to isolate the stretch in the hamstring.

Seated IT Band

1. Sitting on the ground, with both legs out in front of you, gently pull your right shin toward your chest. Hold this for 15 to 30 seconds, then plant your right foot across your left leg so that your right foot is now on the floor to the left of your left knee.
2. Twist your trunk in the opposite direction—to the right—and place your left elbow on your bent right knee. The first part of the stretch works on your hip extensors, while the latter part stretches your IT band and back.
3. Do both stretches and then switch legs.

Lower Back Stretch

1. Lie on your back with your right knee drawn up toward your chest.
2. Slowly swing the bent leg across your body until a stretch is felt in the lower back and hip area. Hold and repeat on the other side.
3. Remember to keep your shoulders squared and flat on the ground at all times. The bottom leg should be straight.

There are many other stretches we can do, but these are the main ones I perform personally.

The thing you want to remember is that stretching is for developing flexibility and preventing injuries—not for losing weight—and it does not count toward your exercise time. You can't spend thirty minutes stretching and then say, "Oh, I worked out for thirty minutes." No, you spent thirty minutes in preventative maintenance. That does not count toward losing weight.

H.I.T. EXAMPLES

Any exercise can become an interval workout. I'm going to include a few examples here that I have used in my own life. But first, some general guidelines, and as I've said before, always see your physician before you start any rigorous exercise routine.

Every workout should begin with a five-minute warm-up that gets your heart rate elevated into your aerobic range and should include a five-minute cooldown at the end of the workout. This leaves forty to fifty minutes of good hard work per hour-long session.

For each "up" interval, you need to change the setting on your machine or speed at which you work out. Change the resistance, change the speed, or adjust the incline to work out harder. If you're not using machines, then you are simply going to go faster. A period of all-out effort for your "up" interval is best. For each "down" interval, you want to lower those same settings until you're back in your aerobic heart rate range.

Here is a sample of an interval routine on an elliptical machine, followed by several other routines. The elliptical is a good way to get in a strenuous workout, especially for people looking for something a little more low impact on the knees. The first column is the time; the second column represents the difficulty or the resistance level of the machine. Your elliptical machine or treadmill may have a different range of levels, so try to follow the general pattern here if you can't use the numbers exactly.

Pete's Elliptical Workout

Warm-up	
Minute 00:00–05:00	Level 3
Workout	
Minute 05:00–06:00	Level 5
Minute 06:00–07:00	Level 10
Minute 07:00–09:00	Level 6
Minute 09:00–11:00	Level 11
Minute 11:00–14:00	Level 7
Minute 14:00–17:00	Level 12
Minute 17:00–21:00	Level 8
Minute 21:00–25:00	Level 13
Minute 25:00–30:00	Level 9
Minute 30:00–35:00	Level 14
Minute 35:00–40:00	Level 10
Minute 40:00–45:00	Level 15
Minute 45:00–50:00	Level 11
Minute 50:00–55:00	Level 16
Cooldown	
Minute 55:00–60:00	Level 3

Here are some more cardio routines, both intervals and steady state.

CARDIO INTERVALS

Beginning 1 Intervals (any machine)	
5 minutes	Warm-up
:30 seconds	Up interval (at aerobic max and above)
4:30 minutes	Down interval (within aerobic range)
Next 50 minutes	Repeat
5 minutes	Cooldown
Beginning 2 Intervals (any machine)	
5 minutes	Warm-up
1 minute	Up interval (at aerobic max and above)
4 minutes	Down interval (within aerobic range)
Next 50 minutes	Repeat
5 minutes	Cooldown
Intermediate Intervals (any machine)	
5 minutes	Warm-up
1 minute	Up interval (at aerobic max and above)
2 minutes	Down interval (within aerobic range)
Next 50 minutes	Repeat
5 minutes	Cooldown

**PETE'S TREADMILL WORKOUT (ALL WALKING)—NO HOLDING ON!
(MODIFY FOR YOUR MACHINERY)**

Warm-up	
2 minutes	Speed 3.5 or so—Incline 2
2 minutes	Speed 3.5 or so—Incline 4
Workout	
2 minutes	Speed 3.5 or so—Incline 6
2 minutes	Speed 3.5 or so—Incline 8
2 minutes	Speed 3.5 or so—Incline 10
2 minutes	Speed 3.5 or so—Incline 12
2 minutes	Speed 3.5 or so—Incline 15
Repeat 5 times for a total of 50 minutes	
Cooldown	
2 minutes	Speed 3.5 or so—Incline 6
2 minutes	Speed 3.5 or so—Incline 4
2 minutes	Speed 3.5 or so—Incline 2
2 minutes	Speed 3.5 or so—Incline 0

KICK BUTT ELLIPTICAL WORKOUT—STRAIGHT FROM *THE BIGGEST LOSER* RANCH

(This is for a Precor Elliptical 576i with incline *and* resistance. Modify for your machinery.)

Incline	Resistance	RPM	Time	Direction
10	10	100	10 minutes	Forward
10	10	90	10 minutes	Reverse
10	18	100	10 minutes	Forward
10	18	90	10 minutes	Reverse
5	3	120	10 minutes	Reverse
5	3	120	10 minutes	Forward

PETE'S FINAL MONTH INTERVAL WORKOUT
Highly Advanced!

1-hour incline sprints 2x per week
Incline 12 / Speed 10
2 minutes sprinting / 1 minute rest
Repeat for 1 hour
Fall over dead. Call ambulance.

STEADY STATE CARDIO EXAMPLES

PETE'S A.M. TREADMILL WORKOUT

Warm-up (modify for your machinery)	
5 minutes	HR 70 to 80% (Speed 5.0 or so—Incline 1)
Workout	
25 minutes	HR 80 to 85% (Speed 5.5 or so—Incline 2)
25 minutes	HR 85 to 95% (Speed 6.5 or so—Incline 2)
Cooldown	
5 minutes	HR 70—80% (Speed 5.0 or so—Incline 1)

PETE'S "MIDNIGHT 20" TREADMILL WORKOUT

Warm-up (modify for your machinery)
2 minutes
Speed 5.0 or so—Incline 1 (HR 70 to 85%)
Workout
15 minutes
Speed 7.5 or so—Incline 2 (HR 85 to 95%)
Warm down
3 minutes
Speed 4.5 or so—Incline 1 (HR 70 to 85%)

For more workout resources, check out www.PeteThomas.com.

MAXIMUM RETURN

Your body contains four types of fat. The types and functions of each are not as important here as actually getting rid of the excess subcutaneous fat. The question is: How do you get rid of it? How can you get the maximum fat-burning return on your exercise investment? You really can maximize your investment, and over the next few chapters I will show you how.

Studies show that when it comes to cardiovascular exercise, steady state is good, but high-intensity interval training (H.I.I.T.) is better. In the next chapter, I'll explain about the different types of resistance training and how incorporating them can improve your weight loss even more. Optimal fat loss requires a combination of different types of workouts. We introduce this magic formula in the next chapter. Remember our F.I.T.T. model:

Frequency + Intensity + Time + Type = Your Result

Your result is always going to be to Lose It Forever. But how quickly do you want to lose it? That's what you need to decide.

KEY POINTS

- Cardiovascular exercise uses the largest muscles in the body—the legs—to work the heart and lungs and pull the fat out of the rest of the body.
- With correct intensity, steady state can burn a great deal of calories during exercise.
- Studies show that when it comes to cardiovascular exercise, steady state is good, but high-intensity interval training (H.I.I.T.) is better.
- To deal with pain, you've got to work through it, work around it, or wrap it up.

CHAPTER 11 CHALLENGES

Create a Road Map to Success

Write down the answers to these questions in your LIF2 Success Journal to help you build your Road Map to Success:

PART 1—CALORIE INTAKE

What is my Personal Daily Fuel Goal? _____

PART 2—EXERCISE DETAILS

What is my maximum HR? _____

What is my aerobic range? _____ to _____

PART 3—KICK IN THE CARDIO

How much weight do I want to lose long-term? _____

How much time will I commit to a daily workout? _____

Am I truly committed and making this a priority in my life? Yes or No

Begin Steady State Cardio Workouts

In Chapter 1, I asked you to start walking if you had not been exercising at all. Now I'm asking you to start serious aerobic exercise for weight loss twice a week, which hopefully will be the basis of your Perfect Personalized Forever Workout Plan (Chapter 13). With this in mind, this week I want you to complete two sixty- to ninety-minute steady state cardio workouts within your aerobic range, which again is 75 to 85 percent of your maximum heart rate. You can use any of the types of cardio exercise mentioned in this chapter.

Begin H.I.I.T. Cardio Workouts

Complete two sixty-minute high-intensity interval training (H.I.I.T.) cardio workouts at or above the upper end of your aerobic range (85 percent) this week. You can use one of the examples in this chapter. Continue to do these twice weekly until you get to Chapter 13, at which point you will be building your own Perfect Personalized Workout Plan or following one of the plans I have included.

"I am amazed at how much I have improved in my endurance and strength since starting LIF2. For me, gaining weight has been a gradual increase as I have aged. I just needed a push to make myself more active, and I now do six hours of exercise a week. I have lost around 10 pounds since I started, but I have really toned up and lost inches. I am no longer out of breath when going up four flights of stairs at the school I work at, which I do about six times each day."

—KATHE, LIF2 STUDENT

CHAPTER

12

BUILD REAL MUSCLE WITH RESISTANCE TRAINING

HAVE YOU EVER TRIED TO EXERCISE WITH A PERSON LITERALLY ON your back? I have. On *The Biggest Loser* Ranch, if there was ever a point where Jillian thought that we were taking it easy, she would add her own body weight to ours. She actually jumped on my back a few times over the course of my stay on the ranch. But I have to tell you, after about a month or so, when she jumped on my back, she felt no bigger than a Twinkie. I remember thinking to myself, "Woman, I've had meals bigger than you."

We did other workouts that involved moving weight around. One time we worked out near Venice Beach, California. Despite what you're thinking, it was not cool and it was not sexy. We were going for a workout, so it was not fun at all. First we had to walk through the sand, carrying large branches over our heads—and I mean *large* branches. Actually, we were doing isometric exercises, but of course we didn't know that at the time. The branches look a lot cooler than plain barbells, but there was a simple purpose to it—we were working our muscles.

Another not-so-fun activity we did was walk down the beach pulling truck tires through the sand behind us. Imagine this—the more we pulled that truck tire along, the more that tire would sink down in the sand, so the more difficult it became. That's a great example of a progression, which we will talk about later in this chapter. Over time, if we looked like we were doing that activity a little too easily, Jillian would either come stand on the truck tire herself or she would have one of our teammates sit on that tire while we were pulling it through the sand. That meant that the tire would get heavier and heavier to the point where we could barely move the thing. I remember one of my more emotional teammates actually crying during this exercise because he could not move the tire through the sand. In my mind I was thinking, "Well, that's what's supposed to happen, isn't it?" The exercise was supposed to get progressively difficult until we were not able to do it.

What did all these *Biggest Loser* experiences have in common? They all used the principle of resistance.

BENEFITS OF RESISTANCE TRAINING

In Chapter 11 we dealt with cardiovascular exercise. Now I want to cover another exercise type (the second "T" of the F.I.T.T. strategy): resistance training, or exercise with weights. This type of exercise is simply applying force or resistance to the different muscles in your body in order to increase the strength, size, tone, and endurance of your skeletal muscles.

Effective resistance training involves manipulating different variables:

- repetitions (also known as reps)
- amount of weight
- number of sets you will do
- tempo or speed of the movement
- rest time between sets
- type of weight you lift (machine or free weight)

The specific combination of these variables depends on your individual goals.

The reason we use weight while exercising is that pushing against weight—or resistance—builds or sustains muscle. This is important because muscle is the metabolic engine of the body; the more muscle you have, the more fuel or calories the body will need. Muscle requires more fuel than anything else that is going on in the body.

As we get older, we will require fewer calories. This is because for the majority of us, our muscles will atrophy over time. Resistance training helps minimize this.

Building muscle has another great advantage that many people don't know about. Building muscle helps burn more calories long after the workout is over, if we've done it correctly. That's because muscle building requires fuel, so your body can actually burn calories after your exercise session while it is repairing your sore muscles.

And then, of course, there are multiple real life applications for resistance training. Many resistance exercises simulate real life activity. So in a very real way, resistance training can decrease injuries from everyday activities.

To illustrate this, I want to explain how a dead lift works. A dead lift is an exercise where your feet are shoulder-width apart; you bend over and grab weight in the form of dumbbells or a barbell and then stand up erect. This strengthens the muscles in your lower back, the erector spinae muscle group along your spine, and your glutes (or butt muscles).

This movement simulates an activity you're going to do on a regular basis, whether you bend over to pick up a child, lift a bag of groceries, or bend down to pull something from underneath the sink. You are going to use those back muscles on an everyday basis, so strengthening them is going to help you do these tasks easily throughout life without injuring yourself.

RESISTANCE TRAINING GOALS

You can get different results from resistance training, depending on what your goals are. To fashion a proper resistance workout, you have to keep your goals in mind. For instance, is your goal maximum strength? If so, you're going to look similar to an Olympic lifter or a power lifter. If you've ever seen some of these Olympic lifters or power lifters, they are built for maximum strength. They are not interested in building every single muscle group like bodybuilders, just those muscles that maximize their lifting strength.

Or maybe you're looking to build muscle size and definition like a bodybuilder. The goal of bodybuilders is to build the size and definition of every muscle, so they spend long hours highlighting just a single muscle. The typical way that these groups train is to stay on one piece of equipment for a long time. They finish a set, then rest, then finish another set and then rest again. For instance, there's something called a five-by-five program; if you were looking to get your chest really big, you would lie on a flat bench and lift a very heavy weight—almost the maximum weight you could possibly lift—for five reps. Then you would rest for five minutes and then come back and lift that same weight five more times, then rest for five more minutes. You would repeat this five times total. That is not the workout for us because we have different goals, building muscle for health and fitness, not for competitions.

For us, the goal of resistance training is to Lose It Forever and to become what I call "modern-day athletes." In my mind, a modern-day athlete is a person who works and has a family and is healthy enough to participate in a variety of physical activities.

I want you to be able to go on vacation and hike with your family all day in the Grand Canyon, go back to the hotel, get something to eat, take a quick twenty-minute nap, and then go dancing all night with that special someone. Or I want you to be able to go out and do a triathlon just because you can, and then go sightseeing in the evening. Or maybe you just want to get up, work out hard on a Saturday morning, and then go shopping when it's all over. That is what I consider a modern-day athlete. I don't mean someone who is a full-time athlete but someone who participates in athletics or athletic activities on a regular basis to stay healthy.

We want to lose weight, but we also want to be physically fit. I know people who achieve weight loss but are unhealthy because they have not incorporated exercise into their daily lives. Some people who lose weight from surgery fall into this category—okay, they lost some weight, but are they fit enough to participate in physical activities that they couldn't do before? Not likely, because they have not built any muscle.

Since our goal is weight loss and fitness, we have to make sure the type of resistance training we are doing is complementing our goals.

TYPES OF RESISTANCE TRAINING

There are different ways that you can apply resistance to your body to get results. You can use simple body weight if you don't have access to weights. Then there are bands and balls that provide resistance. You can use machine weights or free weights, either at home or at the gym.

Here's another interesting thing about resistance exercises: Every exercise has a progression and a regression. Let's say that we want to work the chest muscles. We want to do a push-up, but when we start out we aren't able do one. What we'll do is regress to an easier form of the exercise. We start off doing a wall push-up, which is just a push-up against the wall. Then we'll progress from the wall to a table and do a table push-up. When that starts to get easy, we'll move to a modified push-up, where you do a push-up from your knees on the floor. Then we would do a standard or a straight push-up. We could make it even harder by doing a push-up using bands or balls. Finally, we will have progressed enough to do a chest press on a machine or a chest press with free weights. Like everything else in this program, you can design your own progressive workout until you are on your journey to losing it forever.

Over time, your body will adapt to any exercise you throw at it and then it will cease to be effective in building muscle. The key is to use progression, or progressively harder exercises, to overcome your muscles' adaptation. To help with your progression, I want you to start an exercise log. You can start one right in your LIF2 Success Journal. It's important for you to track your weight and your progression in this exercise log. This is part of your Challenge for this chapter, but you should begin now, when you are starting your resistance training.

RESISTANCE FOR WEIGHT LOSS

Even though we're lifting weights to build muscle, we're still keeping an eye on losing weight as well. With that in mind, the main indicator of an effective weight loss routine will be your heart rate. That means you've got to exercise in a way that gets your heart rate up, even while doing resistance training. I'll give some examples of this in a minute. Remember that muscle is the engine of the body, and fat is the fuel tank. We want to work our muscles in a way that pulls the fat out of the rest of the body.

When it comes to maximum weight loss, the best type of resistance training is high-intensity circuit resistance training. High-intensity circuit resistance training is two or more exercises performed back-to-back in which you move between the exercises without any rest. The "high-intensity" part of the name means the same as it does in the high-intensity interval training we talked about in the last chapter—we work hard and raise our heart rate as we perform our sets.

We're going to perform each exercise for a certain number of repetitions, say fifteen reps, or for a specific period of time (such as one minute). After that we will move to the next exercise with little or no rest in between. Once a circuit of several different exercises is complete, we may repeat that circuit two or three times before moving to the next circuit. Typically we will perform four to six circuits per workout. Chapter 13 has some good examples. We want to keep moving because we want to elevate the heart rate.

This was one of the secrets to our success on *The Biggest Loser*. Even while we were doing resistance training, we were elevating our heart rate as much and as often as we possibly could. So again, our goal is not simply to build muscle like a regular exerciser or a bodybuilder—that just maximizes muscle gain. Instead we want to exercise in a fashion that builds muscle without hindering weight loss. In the next section, I will introduce you to one of our *Biggest Loser* secrets that helped me lose so much weight on my way to winning the $100,000 prize in Season 2. I lost 195 pounds total and put on 10 pounds of muscle for 185 pounds net—this was based on various tests to determine body fat percentage and muscle mass. Learning the ABCs of circuit resistance training will allow you to lose a great deal in a short amount of time as well.

THE ABCS OF FAT BURNING

So far we have discussed cardiovascular exercise and resistance training. Now it's time to put the two together. To really maximize your workout, you need to combine resistance training and cardiovascular exercise during each and every workout.

Why? Because this builds muscle without slowing your weight loss. We do this through something I call the ABCs of High-Intensity Circuit Resistance Training, where each circuit consists of three exercises:

A   Above the waist
B   Below or at the waist
C   Cardio exercise

Here's an example:

A   Above the waist   Push-ups—1 minute
B   Below or at the waist   Squats—1 minute
C   Cardio exercise   Mountain climbers—1 minute

So real simply, imagine doing one minute of push-ups and then one minute of squats and then one minute of mountain climbers. You want to do each of these back-to-back. Then go back: Do one more minute of push-ups, one more minute of squats, and one more minute of mountain climbers, and then do it again. You're going to do everything in one circuit three times through and then go on to the next circuit. Remember that the amount of time (remember the first "T" of F.I.T.T.?) you spend doing this will help you reach your forever goals.

I prefer this ABC method because one muscle group is resting while another muscle group is working. This allows each muscle time to recover so that it can be pushed hard once again during the next round. Our goal is not to fatigue the muscle but to work it out in an intense fashion over and over to achieve muscle endurance and weight loss by keeping the heart rate elevated.

It's also been theorized that you'll actually burn more calories using the ABCs because of a nerdy principle I learned called PHA, which stands for peripheral heart action. The reason we go from above the waist to below the waist is this principle of PHA. This principle was popularized by a former Mr. Universe who wanted to increase the efficiency of his workouts. It is believed that because the blood first has to start assisting in the work done above the waist and then the blood has to go down to the area below the waist, more calories will be burned during this process. That's why we do it in this fashion. The reason we do cardio is because we want to keep the heart rate elevated as much as possible for maximum weight loss.

HOW MUSCLE IS BUILT

Let me explain how we build muscle. This will help motivate you when the workouts get difficult. As you apply resistance to the muscle, micro-tears form in the muscle, and those micro-tears are then filled in with amino acids and proteins. Once the amino acids and proteins fill in that area, you've got a larger muscle. The work that's done when amino acids and proteins fill in that space takes place after your workout has ended. That's why it's important not to work the same muscles every day. The neat part about this, as I mentioned before, is that your body's energy is required to build the muscle. You will actually be burning calories after your exercise session while it is repairing your sore muscles.

So how heavy should our weights be? We definitely do not want to go light on the weights. We want to pick a weight that we can lift with good form for a maximum number of fifteen reps per set. Or if the set goes for a specified time rather than a certain number of reps, we need to choose a weight we can lift with good form for that time period. Whenever we can lift more than the maximum reps or specified time, we need to add weight—that's called progression.

Our goal should be muscle fatigue. In other words, we want to really tire the muscle out. We don't want to work the muscle to failure—where it can't lift the weight—but we do want to work the muscle until it is tired. That's because we want to really build that muscle along the way. Because the muscle is actually built during the recovery step, you need to give your muscles time to relax. That's why we typically concentrate on each muscle twice a week.

SHOULD WOMEN WORRY ABOUT BULKING UP?

I often hear women say they want a firm, toned appearance but they don't want to "bulk up" or get big. One thing you need to remember is that women typically do not produce enough testosterone to get really huge muscles. Very few women can achieve the look of a Ms. Universe without the help of steroids. Remember, ladies, there is a very important reason we want to build muscle besides a firm, toned appearance—we want muscle on our bodies because we want to burn extra fuel. Muscle is the metabolic engine of the body, so everyone—male and female—wants muscle on the body. Our goal is to work out for athletic performance, and women should not worry about looking like the Hulk.

BALANCE AND AGILITY

All of our resistance workouts on *The Biggest Loser* had multiple purposes. We were working on strengthening specific muscle groups, but also indirectly on agility and balance. One of my exercises was to push against Dr. Jeff to see if we could push each other off the spot on which we were standing. That worked the muscles in our arms and legs, but it also improved our core and balance. That exercise also provided humor because we would often slip and the other person would fall flat on his chest—without injury, of course, as we had hundreds of pounds of padding!

Our workouts will also have multiple purposes. We will be working on strength, agility, balance, speed, and quickness by working our stabilizing muscles indirectly as we're working specific muscle groups. I don't know if you'll ever find yourself on the U.S. Olympic team, but you will find yourself becoming a more balanced and agile person through these workouts.

EMBRACE THE SORENESS

I want to finish this chapter by saying something again—you will experience muscle pain when you start doing resistance. But remember your goal. Once you've lost that last pound that you want to Lose Forever, you're going to look and feel like a new person. So embrace that soreness when you wake up the day after the workout, because you're on your way to a healthier, toned, sexier you!

KEY POINTS

- Resistance training is applying force or resistance to the different muscles in our bodies in order to increase the strength, size, tone, and endurance of our skeletal muscles.
- Every exercise has a progression and a regression to fit the needs of each person; we use regression when an exercise is too hard, and progression when it becomes too easy.
- The main indicator of an effective weight loss routine will be your heart rate, which means you've got to exercise in a way that gets your heart rate up, even while doing resistance training. We do this by following the ABCs: A—Above the waist, B—Below or at the waist, and C—Cardio exercise.

CHAPTER 12 CHALLENGES

New Challenges | Begin Resistance Training

The workout plans in Chapter 13 and Chapter 17 will help you get started. You can either start the resistance circuits listed, or begin to form your own. But I want you to remember what I said about only concentrating on a muscle twice a week and giving it a day off in between to rest and recover.

Record Your Workouts

Start recording each workout in your own personal exercise log. You can do this in the LIF2 Success Journal, but you need to write down all those variables I mentioned:

- repetitions (also known as reps)
- amount of weight
- number of sets you will do
- tempo or speed of the movement

- rest time between sets
- type of weight you lift (machine or free weight)

As your muscles adapt and you move on to heavier weights and more reps, your log will be proof that you're progressing.

Ongoing Challenges | Continue Your Journal and Review Your Lists

Remember to write in your journal each day and review your Personal Success Statement and Personal Power Goals. And make sure that you talk to your team on a regular basis about how you're doing.

"It was great to lose it quickly because I was able to see results and use them as a motivating factor. After taking LIF2, I know that I have the tools and the ability to not only lose weight but be fit. I'm 41 and have young children, so I need to be around this rock for another 60 years . . . I tell people who are thinking of following LIF2 to 'do it now!' If you wait six months you could have lost 35 pounds. And Pete will motivate you—take one look at Pete's before and after pictures, and you will get motivated. If that guy can do it, you can!"

—RODNEY, LIF2 STUDENT

CHAPTER

13

CREATE YOUR PERFECT PERSONALIZED FOREVER WORKOUT PLAN

"HELP! IT'S AN EMERGENCY! BRING THE GOLF CARTS!"

I was standing a mile from *The Biggest Loser* house, hunched over with my hands on my knees, unable to walk a step farther. I had just taken a grueling four-mile hike up and down a mountain. I was exhausted. And you know the worst part? This was my rest day.

It's true. On our first off day on *The Biggest Loser* Ranch, I remember Jillian telling us, "OK, guys, I want you all to go hike up to the mountain." We asked her how far she wanted us to go. She said, "I want you to go all the way to the top." I remember thinking to myself, "You have got to be kidding me! And it's supposed to be my *off* day. Who goes to the top of a mountain? And I weigh almost 400 pounds." I'm from Detroit, Michigan, a very flat area. As I was growing up, the closest thing we had to a mountain was when a house in the neighborhood was knocked down and got covered over with dirt. We would ride our bicycles up and down that "mountain."

But Jillian told us go hike the mountain, and so off we went. The ranch was located in Simi Valley, California, at the bottom of the mountain we were supposed to hike. Early in the morning we started this trek up the mountain, and we were just going and going and going. I have to tell you, the closer we got to the top of the mountain, the more likely it seemed that we were about to spontaneously combust. I could feel the sun beating down on me and I remember looking ahead of me and thinking, "Oh my goodness, Seth is changing colors. He started off with a gray sweatshirt and now he's got on a red sweatshirt. What is going on?" And then I realized that, no, Seth had just taken off his shirt and was sporting a nasty sunburn.

I kept hearing these noises all around me. I'm a city boy, and before we left we were warned that there were rattlesnakes up on the trails. I can remember at one point I was incredibly scared because I heard this loud noise and I thought it was the largest rattlesnake ever discovered by humankind and it was coming to attack me, and then I looked back and it was a couple of mountain bikers. They were very polite, saying, "Excuse me," as they continued riding on past us.

The hike was torturous. It took us two and a half hours to hike from the bottom of the mountain all the way up to the top, and then another hour and a half to get back down. All the way I thought I was going to die of exhaustion, if I didn't get bitten by a snake first. I asked God on the way down, "Why am I here? This is supposed to be my day off."

Ironically, once we got back to the bottom of the mountain we still had to walk a mile uphill to where the house was. We were so exhausted that we immediately plotted to get some help. We got on these walkie-talkies they had given us for emergencies and acted like we were having one. "Help! Can anybody hear us? Bring some water and come down here immediately—we need help!"

Of course, the production assistants immediately hopped in the golf carts and drove to the bottom of the hill thinking we had fallen off a cliff or something. When they got to the bottom of the hill they asked us,

"What's wrong? Who's hurt?" That's when we fessed up, "Nobody—we're just so tired we can't go another step. Move over, we're all piling in." We grabbed the water bottles they brought and began to chug while the production assistants rode us back up the hill in the golf cart. That was our "off day."

In this chapter, you're going to create your own Perfect Personalized Forever Workout Plan, which will include your own rest day. Hopefully your rest day will not be as strenuous as ours at the ranch, but I do want you to plan activities that keep you moving on that day. Your plan will take into account your goals, your lifestyle needs, and your growing list of Forever Habits.

DEVELOPING YOUR OWN CIRCUIT ROUTINE

In the upcoming pages you will see that I've designed four separate exercise plans to try to accommodate people with a variety of goals and time schedules. The first one, which appears at the end of this chapter, is my Get Off the Couch or Die—Absolute Beginner 6-Week Workout Plan. The purpose of that plan, which includes six weeks of just one type of exercise—walking—is pretty obvious from the title. It will allow someone to ease into an exercise habit while still providing enough intensity to shed those Forever Few pounds. This plan is in response to the many people who come to me and beg me to help them get their life back. I give them this plan and see if they really want to change—or if they are one of those "you-do-it-for-me" dieters I talked about in the Introduction.

Another plan you will find at the end of this chapter is my 20-Minute-a-Day Weekly Workout Plan. This plan is designed for people without a lot of weight to lose who have a very limited amount of time. I tend to be skeptical of people who say they don't have time to exercise, because a lot of times this is just an excuse for not making an effort. But a friend of mine—a female ob-gyn from Atlanta with young children—convinced me that some people truly don't have much "disposable time." This one-week plan works all the major muscle groups intensely and quickly to maintain a minimum level of fitness. This plan is also good for people who travel a lot and don't have access to equipment all the time.

If you want to lose your weight in the quickest and safest possible way—notice I said safe, which would rule out the surgical options—you will find a very effective plan in Chapter 17, my Lose It Fast 12-Week Workout Plan. This plan is very specific and follows all the principles I will teach you in this chapter. People who have a lot to lose and don't want to take multiple years to do it would benefit from this plan, as would someone who wants to lose that last stubborn few before swimsuit season.

The final plan, my Lose It Forever Weekly Maintenance Workout Plan, can be found in Chapter 18. This one-week plan is heavy on the cardiovascular training, with cardio scheduled on Monday, Wednesday, Friday, and Saturday, and circuit resistance training on Tuesday and Thursday. The maintenance plan is for people who have lost their weight but want to keep their Forever Habit of exercise going so they don't gain it back. This plan is also good for runners, who are encouraged by the medical community to include two days of resistance to go along with their three to four days of cardio.

Everybody should find something that meets their needs with this variety of plan. However, it is very important to not just be told what to do but to learn the *why* and *how* of what you are doing as well. Once you go through the workouts I have provided, it would be fairly simple to recycle through them over and over. On the other hand, if you learn how to put together your own circuits and workouts you will be able to make adjustments and tweaks to your circuits and keep your workouts fresh. You will also learn about your body's muscle groups, which will help you identify problem areas in your body that may need additional work. These reasons alone are worth learning how to develop a circuit routine and an entire workout.

If you are not interested in building your own routine and just want to follow the exercises in one of the plans provided, then you can skip to the workout plan of your choice. But before going there, at the very least read the sections below that discuss the front (anterior) and back (posterior) muscle groups. A basic understanding of muscle groups within the circuits will also give you an introduction as to which body parts you are working. That way, whether you're working out alone or with a trainer, you will always know exactly what it is you are doing and what you are trying to accomplish.

GOOD, BETTER, BEST WORKOUTS

This first routine is what I am going to call a "Good" circuit routine. I have already mentioned the importance of having a warm-up. Five minutes of cardio, such as a five-minute jog, plus the stretches I mentioned earlier, should be sufficient. After the warm-up comes an Above the waist exercise, a Below or at the waist exercise, and a Cardio exercise.

If you put a little more work into choosing certain exercises, you can create what I call a "Better" circuit routine. Remember in the last chapter, I told you that we only wanted to work out each muscle a couple of times a week. So when I say you can make a Better routine, what you're going to do is divide the muscles between the front of the body and the back of the body. You're going to work the anterior muscles, which are typically the push muscles on the front of the body, twice a week, on Mondays and Thursdays. And then you're going to do the posterior muscles—which are typically the pull muscles in the back of the body—twice a week on Tuesdays and Fridays.

Most of your anterior, or "push," muscles are in the front of the body:

- shoulders
- chest
- abdomen
- quadriceps
- triceps (a push muscle, even though it's at the back of the arm)

Most of your posterior, or "pull," muscles are in the back of the body:

- upper and lower back
- gluteus (butt)
- hamstrings
- calves
- biceps (a pull muscle, even though it's at the front of the arm)

To begin designing a Better circuit routine, start off by having a five-minute warm-up. Then choose an Above the waist anterior exercise from the "push" list for Monday and Thursday, then a Below the waist anterior exercise, then a Cardio. You get the idea. Write in an A, a B, and a C for your front-of-body days, Monday and Thursday. Actually, I want you to come up with five different circuits to build in some variety. After that, come up with five circuits that include an A, a B, and a C from the "pull" list for your back-of-body days, Tuesday and Friday.

CREATING THE BEST CIRCUITS OF ALL

At this point I'd like to help you create what I call the "Best" circuit routine by adding yet one more layer. You've already divided your muscles into front/back groups. You can further divide your body into two classes of muscles. First you have what they call prime movers—these are the main muscles in the body—and then there are support muscles. For instance, if you're going to do a push-up, the prime muscle that typically gets work is your chest—your pectorals. But you've also got muscles that assist, such as the triceps in the arms.

Here's the problem: If you were to design a workout routine that worked the triceps first and then moved on to the chest—a prime mover— you would not really get a strong workout on this muscle. Why? Because you've weakened those smaller or support muscles and therefore you can't really work the bigger prime muscles as efficiently as possible. That's why we want to frontload our workouts with exercises that work those larger muscles first.

I've given you multiple examples of exactly how to do that. You can see in my Lose It Fast 12-Week Workout Plan in Chapter 17 that I've designed all the ABC Circuits this way. In week 1, for example, your "A" exercises begin with the chest, then move down to the quads, and end with the biceps. By doing it in this fashion, we are able to work the larger muscles and then those support muscles.

Now using the exercises in this chapter or Chapter 17, I want you to create your own set of six circuits. Make them your Best ABC Circuits so that you can work those large muscles first and then come back and work the smaller muscles on your way to losing that Forever Few. You can find a list of exercises and their descriptions following the Lose It Fast 12-Week Workout Plan in Chapter 17.

FOLLOWING THE PLAN

If you don't want to create your own exercise program, you can use any of the plans I've included in this chapter, depending on how much time you want to spend and your goals. As I explain how to perform the circuits, I'm going to use the Lose It Fast 12-Week Workout Plan as an example.

You will see that each circuit day contains six circuits. The circuit days are Monday, Tuesday, Thursday, and Friday. On Monday and Thursday you will work your front, or anterior, muscles, and on Tuesday and Friday you will work your back, or posterior, muscles. The circuits are also arranged so that your larger muscles are worked first, then the small, supporting muscles follow later. This makes each workout most efficient. In addition, the exercises change every two weeks to get progressively more demanding as the weeks progress.

I want you to do all the exercises in the circuit for one minute each. (See the next section to learn how to modify an exercise if it is too difficult for you.) Go through each circuit three times before you move on to the next circuit. You can rest for fifteen seconds between each exercise within the circuit, and after you complete your three times through the circuit, rest for one full minute before moving on to the next circuit. So the example I used before will look something like this:

A Above the waist   Push-ups—1 minute
    (rest 15 seconds)

B Below or at the waist   Squats—1 minute
    (rest 15 seconds)

C Cardio exercise   Mountain climbers—1 minute
    (rest 15 seconds)

Repeat circuit a second time
    (rest 15 seconds)

Repeat circuit a third time
    (rest 1 full minute)

Move on to circuit #2

You don't need a gym membership to do the exercises in this book, but some of the exercises require some basic equipment. You will need a set of heavy dumbbells (I usually recommend women start with 10-, 15-, and 25-pound weights, and men start with 15-, 20-, and 30-pound weights), and of course a good pair of shoes!

MODIFYING THE CIRCUITS FOR BEGINNERS

Lose It Fast, Lose It Forever can be adapted to any life situation and any level of experience. If these exercises are too difficult for you at first, don't worry—you can modify them in two simple ways.

The first modification will be the time duration of each exercise. I want you to eventually do each exercise in each circuit for one minute. If that is too long a duration at first, you can work out in *ascending increments*, meaning you can start at thirty seconds for twelve weeks, then progress to forty-five seconds for twelve weeks, and so on until you reach one minute per exercise. Once you reach the one-minute mark, don't cheat and go back, because you will burn fewer and fewer calories as your body adapts to the workout.

The second way to make the circuits a little easier is to do fewer of the circuits listed on a particular day. You'll still do each circuit three times for the same duration, but instead of doing all six in one day, you can do the following:

- The first four circuits for 47 minutes—Basic Level
- The first five circuits for 59 minutes—Intermediate Level
- All six circuits for 71 minutes—Advanced Level

When you look at the program you will notice that the sixth circuit on every day is all cardio. I call that the Fabulous Finish because that last bit of cardio is going to burn fat like crazy so you will look absolutely fabulous in no time!

YOUR PERFECT PERSONALIZED FOREVER WORKOUT

Now we're going to put it all together and lay out a perfect routine the way that I learned it myself. This is the way I was able to lose 185 pounds in nine months and win $100,000. I call it Your Perfect Personalized Forever Workout Plan. You are going to plan out your entire week—what exercises you are going to do on what days.

On Monday, Tuesday, Thursday, and Friday I recommend that you do your Best ABC weight loss circuits. For maximum fat burning, add an extra cardio segment on top of your ABCs for a Fabulous Finish when time permits. You can find a list of exercises, along with a description, following the Lose It Fast 12-Week Workout Plan in Chapter 17.

On Wednesday and Saturday, I recommend that you have an all-cardio day. Chapter 11 contains some good suggestions for this day, and you can do a combination of high-intensity intervals or steady state cardio. But let's make sure that we have an all-cardio day on Wednesday and then come back and do it again on Saturday. A perfect way to exercise on those days would be a spin class at the gym, going for a jog, riding your bike, something like that. Your rest day is going to be on Sunday if at all possible. But when I say rest day, I don't mean *total* rest.

ACTIVE REST DAYS

You may have caught this from the story at the beginning of the chapter— while I was at *The Biggest Loser* Ranch, Jillian let us know that we were expected to have an active rest day. An active rest day is different than the rest day you're used to right now. Now when I take a full rest day, it looks like my pre–*Biggest Loser* Super Bowl Sunday.

On Super Bowl Sunday I'm going to make it to church and then I'm coming straight home. Once I come home I don't want to be bothered by anyone—I've got my "triangle of relaxation" going on. That triangle consists of three locations: the first is right on the sofa in front of the game; then there is a line that goes over to the kitchen; and the third is a line that goes straight to the bathroom. I'm triangulating my position so that I am in the center of all of those positions. I'm looking at the television, I'm walking to the kitchen to get some snacks, and I'm going to the bathroom, then back to the sofa.

That is my idea of a complete and total rest day. I'm not doing anything—don't ask me—I'm not even reaching too far to pick up the phone unless it's to call a buddy and yell about that last play or to invite him to watch the game with me.

An active rest day is quite different from that. On an active rest day we take the kids to a museum or the zoo, or we may go shopping. We're playing soccer in the yard or gardening. We're walking around and being active, although we are not elevating our heart rate too much or taxing specific muscle groups. We're active on a rest day because that's part of losing it forever—keeping our bodies moving because we want to, not because we have to through a workout.

MAXIMUM FAT LOSS, ANYONE?

Keep in mind the F.I.T.T. formula: your Frequency plus Intensity plus Time plus Type equals your results. Steady state cardio training is good, but high-intensity interval training cardio is even better. Resistance training is good, but circuit resistance training is better. And of course, the absolute best way to accomplish your fat loss goals, in my opinion, is high-intensity circuit resistance training (the ABCs). That's the method that I use. Optimal fat loss requires a combination of these different workouts.

At the beginning of this program, you probably wondered how you would lose the weight you want to lose. Now that you've learned about both nutrition and the various kinds of exercise, is losing it fast and losing it forever looking more doable? It should, because you are well on your way to reaching all your weight loss goals!

PETE THOMAS'S GET OFF THE COUCH OR DIE—ABSOLUTE BEGINNER 6-WEEK WORKOUT PLAN

Frequency   6 weeks, 5 to 6 days per week
Intensity   Any elevation of your maximum heart rate
Time   30 to 55 minutes per day
Type   Walking / Cardio (time-focused—ignore speed and distance)

	Monday	Tuesday	Wednesday	Thursday	Friday	Saturday	Sunday
WEEK 1	30 minutes Walking / Cardio	30 minutes Walking / Cardio	Active Rest Day	30 minutes Walking / Cardio	30 minutes Walking / Cardio	30 minutes Walking / Cardio	Active Rest Day
WEEK 2	35 minutes Walking / Cardio	35 minutes Walking / Cardio	Active Rest Day	35 minutes Walking / Cardio	35 minutes Walking / Cardio	35 minutes Walking / Cardio	Active Rest Day
WEEK 3	40 minutes Walking / Cardio	40 minutes Walking / Cardio	40 minutes Walking / Cardio	40 minutes Walking / Cardio	40 minutes Walking / Cardio	40 minutes Walking / Cardio	Active Rest Day
WEEK 4	45 minutes Walking / Cardio	45 minutes Walking / Cardio	45 minutes Walking / Cardio	45 minutes Walking / Cardio	45 minutes Walking / Cardio	45 minutes Walking / Cardio	Active Rest Day
WEEK 5	50 minutes Walking / Cardio	50 minutes Walking / Cardio	50 minutes Walking / Cardio	50 minutes Walking / Cardio	50 minutes Walking / Cardio	50 minutes Walking / Cardio	Active Rest Day
WEEK 6	55 minutes Walking / Cardio	55 minutes Walking / Cardio	55 minutes Walking / Cardio	55 minutes Walking / Cardio	55 minutes Walking / Cardio	55 minutes Walking / Cardio	Active Rest Day

Tools   Purchase a pair of running shoes from a specialty running store. Buy a heart rate monitor that tracks heart rate and gives a summary of the entire workout. I use a Polar FT7.

Perform standard warm-up and cooldown exercises as necessary.

Notes   The goal is an elevated heart rate, so increase your speed as you progress through the weeks.

PETE THOMAS'S 20-MINUTE-A-DAY WEEKLY WORKOUT PLAN

	Exercise 1	Exercise 2	Exercise 3	Exercise 4	Exercise 5
Monday	Push-ups	Air Squats	Biceps Curls with DB	Sit-ups	Jumping Jacks
Tuesday	1-Arm Row with DB*	Reverse Lunge*	Overhead Triceps Extensions with DB*	Bicycles	High Knees
Wednesday	20 minutes cardio (optional)				
Thursday	Chest Press with DB	Sumo Squats	Biceps Hammer Curls with DB	Planks	Butt Kicks
Friday	High Rows with DB	Forward Lunge*	Triceps Kickbacks with DB	Side Planks*	Up Downs (10 count)

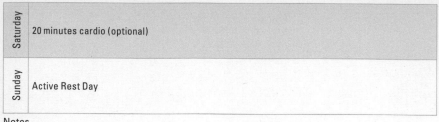

| Saturday | 20 minutes cardio (optional) |
| Sunday | Active Rest Day |

Notes

Perform all exercises Tabata-style: 20 seconds of all-out effort followed by 10 seconds of rest x 8 rounds =
    4 minutes of work per exercise x 5 exercises = 20 minutes per day.
DB = dumbbell. Bands can be substituted for dumbbells.
* = Rotate positions after 4 rounds when necessary. For example: Perform a row with the right arm for 4 rounds
    and then switch to the left arm for 4 rounds.
Perform lunges on the right leg for 4 rounds and then switch to the left leg for 4 rounds.
Perform overhead triceps extensions with the right side for 4 rounds and then switch to the left side for 4 rounds.
Perform side planks on the right side for 4 rounds and then switch to the left side for 4 rounds.
Perform standard warm-up and cooldown exercises as necessary.

KEY POINTS

■ To really maximize your workout, you need to use the ABCs of High-Intensity Circuit Resistance Training:
  • A—Above the waist
  • B—Below or at the waist
  • C—Cardio exercise
■ To be as efficient as possible, we want to frontload our workouts with exercises that work those larger muscles first.
■ Your rest day is going to be on Sunday—but it is an *active* rest day.

CHAPTER 13 CHALLENGES

New Challenges | Create Your Perfect Personalized Forever Workout Using Your Own Personalized Circuits

Write down your "Best" exercise routines from the examples in this chapter or Chapter 17. You will find descriptions of all the exercises in my plans in Chapter 17, after the Lose It Fast 12-Week Workout Plan. Remember to leave at least one rest day between working the different muscles in your body.

Or Start Using the Plans Here or in Chapter 17

Begin following either a plan from this chapter or the Lose It Fast 12-Week Workout Plan in Chapter 17. If some exercises are too difficult at first, remember to use a modification that is easier.

Alternate Cardio and ABC Circuits

Declaring Wednesday and Saturday as all-cardio days is a good idea if you are doing resistance circuits on Monday, Tuesday, Thursday, and Friday. You'll be burning calories and shedding fat while resting your muscles. You'll find good suggestions in Chapter 11.

Ongoing Challenges | Continue Recording Your Workouts

Hopefully you've been recording each workout in your LIF2 Success Journal. If not, start right now!

"I am training for a half marathon in May. Yesterday I went 12 miles and followed it with a 2½-hour yoga workshop. My energy has increased so much I barely recognize myself. I think often we get too focused on weight and not enough on long-term health, which is why the bulk of my goals concern changes in my physical, mental, and social health. I have met all these goals. However, as of this morning, I have also lost 50.6 pounds."

—JENNIFER, LIF2 STUDENT

CHAPTER

RUNNING IS FOR WINNERS

ON JULY 4, 2005, I PARTICIPATED IN ANN ARBOR'S ANNUAL 5K RUN. You may not think this is such a big deal. Maybe you've run a 5K before, but I hadn't. I was running my first one—at a svelte 302 pounds. I was ecstatic just to be in that environment that morning. I was surrounded by all these little people. Runners. And I was slowly but surely becoming one of them. I had come to that realization a month before in the middle of a rainstorm, but I will get to that story in a little bit.

Not only was my first 5K very memorable to me; it was very fulfilling as well. I ran that race nonstop at 302 pounds and then the very next day I ran for over two hours straight on the treadmill. How was I able to do this? I had reached a goal I had set for myself even before I was cast on *The Biggest Loser*—I had learned *how* to run.

AN EXERCISE THAT'S MORE THAN AN EXERCISE

I was sent home from *The Biggest Loser* late in the spring of 2005. Over that summer I learned something that changed my life—how to run. I made the decision to join a beginner's running group, and I'm glad I did. The group taught me to run in a way that was not only safe but effective for a person of my size. This was instrumental not just in losing weight fast but losing it forever. That's something I want to get across to you— not everybody knows how to run properly. A lot of people think about sprinting as fast as they can when they think of running. That's not what we're going to do. There is a specific quantifiable difference between running all-out for distance (three miles, for example) and running for time. I want you to understand that we're going to be running for time. Don't worry, I will explain what I mean by that in a minute.

The objective of this chapter is to introduce you to running, biking, and swimming for weight loss and weight maintenance. I will spend the majority of the chapter talking about running. We will explore the different types of running methods for beginners and emphasize heart rate training as made popular by Dr. Phil Maffetone. I'm also going to explain the three main energy systems—aerobic, anaerobic, and VO_2 max.

Now right off the top you may be thinking, "I don't want to run, it's too hard." And it's true; it is hard at first. But running pays huge dividends in weight loss and maintenance, so at least hear me out before you move on. After all, I attribute at least 70 pounds of the 185 pounds that I lost directly to learning to run. So it's important that you keep reading.

THE BENEFITS OF RUNNING

Running has a lot of benefits, which is what drove me to want to learn how to do it properly. One benefit is that running can be done just about anywhere. People run in deserts, in Antarctica, in big cities, and on ships in the middle of the ocean. This is important if you travel or cannot always make it to a gym. Running also requires minimal equipment, as shown by the recent trend in barefoot running—which I do not recommend for you, by the way. Running strengthens the cardiovascular system, helps prevent osteoporosis, and lowers many negative health risk factors.

FROM TORTOISE TO HARE

Even at my largest, I was absolutely set on learning to run. I remember going to my ironically named local running shoe store here in Ann Arbor, Michigan—Tortoise and Hare. I am very thankful that I stumbled upon this particular store because I was matched up with the perfect teammates there in the form of the store's owners, Matt Holappa and Monica Joyce. When I walked through the door at over 400 pounds, Matt didn't look at me like, "Oh, my goodness, what is he doing in here? Does he not realize the bakery is around the corner?" No, he looked at me like I was an actual person, like someone who might one day become a runner.

The very first thing Matt did was to recommend the best shoes for the way I walked and for my weight. When I got to *The Biggest Loser* Ranch approximately one year later (yes, I set a great goal to become a runner long before I ever even applied to the show), I had barely even used those running shoes. Nevertheless, they were perfect for my experience on the ranch. I was able to work out extremely hard without having any foot problems because of the specialized shoes that fit my specific foot type.

As a matter of fact, a majority of the male contestants back in Season 2 struggled with some type of foot or shoe issues. As the contestants began to work out hard and lose weight, many of us ran into foot and shoe problems. At one point, the executive producer got tired of the shoe problems and asked Bob Harper, who was an avid runner, "What type of shoes should all the contestants be in?" Bob looked over at me and said, "Whatever shoe Pete is wearing." As I said earlier in this book, the right shoes are very important. It's worth the time and effort to get them from an actual running store from professionals who will match you with the perfect shoe.

PASSING THE TEST

Once I was voted off the show, I decided to again pursue my goal of becoming a runner. So I went back to my running store and signed up for the beginner's running class. What makes this particular class unique is that they start with absolute beginners. The owner of the store, Matt, is a slim guy who has been a runner all his life. His wife, Monica, is a former

Olympian who currently holds the world record in the mile for women over age 50. Even with all of this professional experience, they were able to work with and teach folk three times their size and with none of their natural talent. This is a rare ability indeed.

I can remember my very first running class. Because of the timing of returning home after being voted off *The Biggest Loser* Ranch, I actually missed the first week of class. As luck would have it, on the day I arrived for my first class, we were scheduled to take a test! I couldn't believe it. A test? In a running class? Yes, we had to take what's called a MAF—or maximum aerobic function—test. The running instructors asked me right away, "Pete, do you want to run one mile or two?" and I said, "Neither! I don't run, I walk."

As a matter of fact, that's mainly what I had done while I was on *The Biggest Loser* Ranch. While we did work out very hard, we didn't actually need to run. That's because Jillian would increase the incline of the treadmill up to a level of 15 and our heart rates would just go through the ceiling. We would get incredible workouts just from the walking. But I wanted and needed to progress from there, and running was the next logical step.

After further prodding by Matt and Monica, I chose to run the one-mile option for my MAF test. I found someone who ran about the same pace that I did (she was twenty years older than me, I believe) and I began to just follow her while keeping my heart rate within the required range. Someone to pace myself with helped me so very much. You probably know that four laps on a track equal one mile, and after about three laps I looked up at Matt and Monica and said, "You know what, I think I can finish this mile and even go another mile." And that's exactly what I did. I kept my heart rate within range and I kept pressing on and on and on and somehow I completed two miles nonstop. It was so amazing. I couldn't wait for the class to end so that I could call some friends and tell them I had run two miles nonstop for the first time in my life.

Now mind you, at this time I was still was around 318 pounds, but I was ecstatic about being able to run that far nonstop. That was how I started my love affair with running, even though I was still pretty heavy. Running gets easier and more fun as you lose weight and have less to lug around.

MIND OVER BLUBBER

Most likely the biggest barrier to developing a habit of running will involve breaking through the mental barriers in starting out. On many occasions my running class would run at an outdoor track at the University of Michigan, and it would be a struggle just for me to run an entire lap nonstop—even though I had already done it for my MAF test. There was a tree off to one side, right after the start/finish line on this track. Near the end of each lap I would get to this tree and stop running and start walking. It just became a habit. I would start walking as soon as I approached this tree. There was absolutely nothing physically wrong with me and there was no reason not to run the full lap, but every time I approached the tree I literally remember saying to myself, "You should not be running. You are too fat to run." I fought these thoughts every month, every week, every day, and every single lap! My coaches and fellow runners would push me and encourage me to keep going. I would rehearse past success and even would turn up my music player to drown out my thoughts. Eventually, after months of trying, I ran past the mental block that was that tree.

One day my running group was running in a beautiful place called the Arboretum here in Ann Arbor, Michigan, when it started to rain pretty solidly. We were running through a grassy field in the middle of a woodsy area. These surroundings were a far cry from my upbringing in the concrete grounds of the inner city. Prior to this day I would have asked, "Why run through the woods when you can drive around them?" Even on that day as I was running I said to myself, "It's raining pretty hard. I should be in the house on the sofa." But I just kept running because I was with my running group (great teammates are the key to success!) and because I was enjoying it so much. It was at that point that I realized something and said to myself, "I'm not just running; I'm a runner." When I came to that realization, I went ahead and signed up for the 5K I told you about at the beginning of the chapter. That's how it starts. Slowly and steadily, and before you know it you're doing something you have only heard about others doing. It is really an amazing feeling.

GETTING STARTED

When learning to run, I want you to remember a few things. First, you want to stay within your aerobic range. I talked about that in Chapter 10. Our focus when running is on heart rate and time, not on speed and distance. When I say time, I don't mean how fast you finish your mile; I'm talking about the length of time you are exercising or running. For example, we may jog for fifteen, thirty, or even sixty minutes and not care how many miles we cover. This is much different from most approaches and programs that promote running to beginners. Remember, put in the time and the miles will take care of themselves.

If you can, take a beginner's class that focuses specifically on heart rate training. Check out your local running store, like I did, or look for running groups in your area. Every beginner's class is not the same, so make sure to compare programs closely. A good program is one that knows that beginning runners need people to run with and encourage them. A good program will also teach you about gait and form as well as about heart rate training.

I've learned that runners are an unusual group. If you run and you weigh over 200 pounds, they call you a Clydesdale. That's literally how you're listed on the results of many races. That makes me think that runners don't particularly like too many new people within their group. Otherwise they wouldn't call you a giant horse. In my opinion, most programs and even running magazines do a poor job of providing anything of value to the beginning runner, as most writers and editors have been running for a long time. My point is to carefully shop around for a beginner's running class that focuses on heart rate training. If you take a class that is not specifically geared toward you, the discouragement factor could cause you to drop out and miss out on an excellent Forever Habit. So don't just take any old class.

I understand not everybody can take a running class because of finances or location challenges. I have included a mini–beginner's running course in an upcoming section so you can get moving toward your goal of running. But first I want to cover a couple more topics.

RUN-WALK-RUN VERSUS HEART RATE TRAINING

Let me give you a couple of different types of beginning running methods. The first is the Run-Walk-Run method made popular by Jeff Galloway. Basically, as a beginner you would run a minute, walk a minute, run a minute, walk a minute. An intermediate person would run a mile, walk a minute, run a mile, walk a minute. The advanced runner would run at a 10K pace, walk a minute, run at a 10K pace, and then walk a minute, for a specified period of time. If you want more information about this method, see www.jeffgalloway.com.

My preferred method, as I've mentioned, is from Dr. Phil Maffetone. He is one of the pioneers of heart rate training, and he's been doing it for years. One of his famous articles on the subject is "Want Speed . . . Slow Down," which you can find on his website, www.philmaffetone.com. That means you have to actually go slower to get faster. This all came from his experience working with triathletes.

To illustrate, I'll tell you the story of a famous triathlete and Phil Maffetone protégé, Mike Pigg. Every summer, Mike Pigg would bike from his home to his parents' summer home, which happened to be sixty-five miles away and included three large hills along the way. His previous record for getting to the house was three hours and fifteen minutes and his heart rate ranged between 165 and 182 beats a minute. Having expended all his energy, he would arrive in three hours and fifteen minutes and promptly fall down on his parents' lawn completely exhausted. Once he started training with Dr. Maffetone, he lowered the speed at which he rode and his corresponding heart rate. Lo and behold, he completed the ride in three hours and nine minutes instead of three hours and fifteen minutes. Not only did he shorten his time, he felt so good that he went out and rode an additional ten miles just because he felt fresh. Personally, after I get done with a workout that long, I feel like eating a Twinkie.

So what can we learn from Mr. Pigg? Six minutes may not sound like a lot, but it's a huge improvement for an athlete. The point of this story is that by staying within our aerobic heart rate range while learning to run, we can actually get better over time and not wear ourselves out. In Dr. Phil Maffetone's method, you stay in your aerobic heart rate range every single workout until your body adapts.

With my adaptation to Maffetone's method, I want you to focus on staying at the bottom of your aerobic range as you first learn to run. As you get more in shape, you'll stay near the top of your aerobic range. As I explained in Chapter 10, your aerobic range is 75 to 85 percent of your maximum heart rate. As you're just starting out, you will stay near 75 percent, but eventually you're going to work up to 85 percent of your maximum heart rate.

I have adapted my plan from Dr. Maffetone's original heart rate formula. I use a modification of his formula and suggest an aerobic range based on the popular Karvonen heart rate formula (220 minus your age). I have found that the two formulas come within a couple of beats of each other in most cases, so I prefer to use just one formula for the sake of simplicity. However, if you want to use the original formula developed by Dr. Maffetone, then I recommend you check out his website.

Here's an important note: If you reach your aerobic range by walking, then just keep on walking.

It's okay to start out walking, but over time you'll have to pick it up and start running. You'll get a better workout. When I started running in 2005 at over 300 pounds, staying within my aerobic heart rate range meant going very slowly. I remember going to my local high school and running on the track. It was crowded with all types of people, including a walkers' group. I started off doing my heart rate training, just jogging along, and these walkers were going faster than I was. Now that will mess with your psyche. You're running so slowly that walkers are passing you.

But don't get discouraged. Keep running and an amazing thing happens. You start to become more aerobically fit in no time. When you're running, you are actually exerting more effort than walking, even if it's a slow run. Also, you are actually putting some purposeful stress on the ankles and knees and hips. By stressing those joints intentionally, you're actually going to strengthen them. Stick with the running even though it may be slow going at the beginning.

RUNNING PAIN

I hope by now you realize that when you start working out, you will experience some pain. The results are worth it, but there is no such thing as pain-free growth. Learning to run is no exception. So right now I want to talk about how to deal with the pains of running. First of all, whenever you feel discomfort or pain, the first thing that you should do is consult with an expert. Notice I did not say "physician." Talking to your physician is the *second* thing I would do. Here's why I put them in that order.

I realized early on that the people who knew the most about running injuries to the knees and ankles and joints were the experts at my running store or the physical therapist at a specialty clinic. They constantly deal with knee injuries and foot injuries and know just what to do. So whenever I feel something odd, I immediately go to them and ask, "What about this?" and "What about that?" They always check my equipment and my form. If they find a problem with my form they reiterate the basics: Keep your chest up and your shoulders back; don't stare at the ground but keep your gaze at eye level; relax your shoulders and make sure to adjust your gait if necessary so that your heel is not striking the ground first. On the rare occasion that they cannot simply fix the issue right there in the store, they refer me to a physician. More important, they tell me how to direct the physician so he or she understands my goals.

The reason you follow this path is because when you go to your physician and tell him that something hurts, the first thing that he is going to say is, "Well, stop doing what you're doing." Obviously, that is not what we want to do. I've explained before that we have several options when we experience pain: We can wrap it up, work around it, or work through it. We have to explain to the doctor that we do not want to stop, that we are trying to reach our weight loss goals.

I've had to do that several times. I received information from the running expert and then passed it on to the physician. That teamwork has kept me going through some painful events.

BODY ADJUSTMENTS

On one occasion, just one year after leaving *The Biggest Loser,* I was experiencing incredibly severe knee pain. I went to a no-cost runners' clinic hosted by a physical therapist who works with Olympic runners, and he did an assessment. He couldn't find anything wrong, so he told me, "Okay, you need to go to your doctor and ask for a referral to a specialist." So I did that. But in the meantime, I didn't stop running. The pain was really, really bad, but I did not stop. I would run, endure the pain, and then ice down my knee. Then I would repeat that again the next day and the next.

Because of circumstances, it took me a little longer than planned to get into the specialist's office. And lo and behold, by the time I got to his office—it took me about three weeks or so—the knee pain had miraculously gone away. I learned from this experience that sometimes your body just has to adjust to the pounding of running on a hard surface. It was an amazing experience for me. I ended up canceling the referral. I didn't have to worry about spending the extra money or time to see a specialist because my body had adapted.

Remember that as you start running, the body needs time to adjust outdoors if you've been running on a treadmill. You should consider running on different surfaces when you move outside. Obviously, the hardest surface on the body would be concrete. You want to be careful about running on concrete and try to select something a little softer, such as asphalt. Then there's running on dirt or wood chips or a professional track, for instance at your local school.

When you're dealing with the pains of running, you also want to make sure that you consider knee braces and orthotics if you need them. The expert at your running store can suggest good ones, or a doctor who can prescribe them. It's very important that you make sure you have what you need to get through your runs and your workouts.

RUNNING FOR WEIGHT LOSS

Let me contrast a couple of different types of running styles and the benefits. If you look at professional runners, say a marathon runner versus a sprinter, they're very different. A marathon runner is very slight of frame. In the 2008 Olympics, the male marathon champion—who averaged just over five minutes per mile—was five feet four and less than 115 pounds. By contrast, a sprinter is very strongly built. He or she is rock solid and very muscular. That's because they have different goals when it comes to running. A sprinter is going with an all-out effort for a short period of time, whereas a marathoner is running for longer periods of time with less of an effort.

And what is our goal? We are running to both Lose It Forever and to Lose It Fast. As we are beginning to learn to run we want to build what's known as an aerobic base. To do this we never want to drop below our aerobic range. However, we are ultimately going to maximize our weight loss by mixing various running styles and running in three different energy zones. These are the three zones I'm talking about:

- aerobic heart range
- lactate threshold or anaerobic range
- VO_2 max

This is advanced stuff, but the knowledge will help you achieve maximum weight loss and physical fitness.

Running and cycling will improve all three of your main energy systems. First of all, you build your aerobic base by working within your aerobic heart rate range, which means staying between 75 and 85 percent of your maximum heart rate. Distance runners work primarily in their aerobic range. This is the system that you're going to work primarily as you start your running program.

A strong aerobic energy system provides multiple benefits. One, it builds a stronger heart and lungs. The heart is a muscle, and by working it out, you will make it stronger. Having a strong aerobic energy system is going to lower your blood pressure, provide you with more energy, lower a lot of your negative health risk factors, and give you more energy for circuit resistance training.

The next energy system that you improve by running or cycling is your lactate threshold, or your anaerobic range. This occurs when your body begins to buffer lactic acid and running physically becomes hard. Typically this is ten to twenty beats above your aerobic maximum. We want to work in this range as well. You can stay in your anaerobic range for short periods of time, maybe a couple of minutes. This is where you see an Olympian run for a few minutes around a track—it's not quite an all-out sprint, but it elevates your heart more than the aerobic range. You can't hold that lactate threshold for too long, but you can hold it for ten to twenty beats above your aerobic max. These are longer than sprints but nowhere near as long as your distance runs.

The last energy zone is VO_2 max. This is the maximum amount of oxygen that the body can process. VO_2 max is where you run very hard and make an all-out effort. As an example, if you look at a sprinter, he is going to run all-out for a short period of time—probably less than fifteen seconds. So let's just imagine you're running as fast as humanly possible for 100 yards. That's an all-out VO_2 max sprint.

It's important that you work through all three main energy systems when you're trying to lose weight. To determine your maximum heart rate and your aerobic range, make sure you check out the information in Chapter 10. The good news is that you do not have to be an Olympic athlete to perform these workouts. You can work through these three energy systems while running, cycling, or swimming.

PETE THOMAS'S ABSOLUTE BEGINNERS FRIDGE-TO-5K RUNNING PLAN

Frequency   6 weeks, 4 to 5 days per week (Monday/Wednesday/ Thursday/Saturday)
(ideally you will still do resistance training twice a week)
Intensity   75% to 85% of your maximum heart rate
Time   30 to 45 minutes per day
Type   Jog/walk hybrid (time and heart rate focused—ignore speed and distance)

	Frequency	Intensity	Time	Type
Week 1	4 days a week Mon, Wed, Thurs, Sat	75–80% MHR	30 minutes	4 minutes brisk walk 1 minute jog
Week 2	4 days a week Mon, Wed, Thurs, Sat	75–80% MHR	35 minutes	3 minutes brisk walk 2 minutes jog
Week 3	4 days a week Mon, Wed, Thurs, Sat	75–85% MHR	40 minutes	2 minutes brisk walk 3 minutes jog
Week 4	5 days a week Mon, Tues, Thurs, Fri, Sat	75–85% MHR	45 minutes	1 minute brisk walk 4 minutes jog
Week 5	5 days a week Mon, Tues, Thurs, Fri, Sat	80–85% MHR	50 minutes	1 minute brisk walk 5 minutes jog
Week 6	5 days a week Mon, Tues, Thurs, Fri, Sat	80–85% MHR	45 minutes	45 minutes jog

Tools

Purchase a pair of running shoes from a specialty running store. Buy a heart rate monitor that tracks heart rate and gives a summary of the entire workout. I use a Polar FT7.

Notes

You can pick up this running plan at any point by taking this simple test. Go for a slow jog, keeping your heart rate within 75 to 85 percent. Do not worry about how fast you are moving as long as you are maintaining a steady jog. Concentrate on keeping your heart rate within its aerobic zone. Jog as long as you can without stopping. Then pick this running plan up from that week and continue forward.

Your heart rate should average between 75 and 85 percent of your maximum heart rate for the duration of the workout. You can start out all your runs very slowly in your lower aerobic range, 75 percent, allowing for your legs to warm up, and build up into the higher ranges of 80 to 85 percent. Do not exceed your aerobic max on these runs. Your goal is to develop a strong aerobic base and learn to enjoy running. Post-run you may want to ice your joints for fifteen minutes on and fifteen minutes off to help with aches and pains.

Once you can run forty-five minutes without stopping, you will easily be able to run an entire 5K. Run your 5K between 75 and 85 percent of your maximum heart rate and *enjoy* your run.

PETE THOMAS'S PREFERRED BEGINNER FRIDGE-TO-5K RUNNING PLAN

Frequency   8 weeks, 4 to 5 days per week
Intensity   75% to 85% of your maximum heart rate
Time   5 to 45 minutes per day
Type   All jogging

	Frequency	Intensity	Time and Type
Week 0	4 days a week Mon, Wed, Thurs, Sat	75%–80% MHR	5 minutes jog
Week 1	4 days a week Mon, Tues, Thurs, Fri	75%–80% MHR	10 minutes jog
Week 2	4 days a week Mon, Wed, Thurs, Sat	75%–80% MHR	15 minutes jog
Week 3	4 days a week Mon, Wed, Thurs, Sat	75%–80% MHR	20 minutes jog
Week 4	5 days a week Mon, Tues, Thurs, Fri, Sat	75%–80% MHR	25 minutes jog
Week 5	5 days a week Mon, Tues, Thurs, Fri, Sat	75%–85% MHR	30 minutes jog
Week 6	5 days a week Mon, Tues, Thurs, Fri, Sat	75%–85% MHR	35 minutes jog
Week 7	5 days a week Mon, Tues, Thurs, Fri, Sat	80%–85% MHR	40 minutes jog
Week 8	5 days a week Mon, Tues, Thurs, Fri, Sat	80%–85% MHR	45 minutes jog

Tools

Purchase a pair of running shoes from a specialty running store. Buy a heart rate monitor that tracks heart rate and gives a summary of the entire workout. I use a Polar FT7.

Notes

You can pick up this running plan at any point by taking this simple test. Go for a slow jog, keeping your heart rate within 75 percent to 85 percent. Do not worry about how fast you are moving as long as you are maintaining a steady jog. Concentrate on keeping your heart rate within its aerobic zone. Jog as long as you can without stopping. Then pick this running plan up from that week and continue forward.

Your heart rate should average between 75 percent and 85 percent of your maximum heart rate for the duration of the workout. You can start out all your runs very slowly in your lower aerobic range, 75 percent, allowing for your legs to warm up, and build up into the higher ranges, 80 percent to 85 percent. Do not exceed your aerobic max on these runs. Your goal is to develop a strong aerobic base and learn to enjoy running. Post-run you may want to ice your joints for fifteen minutes on and fifteen minutes off to help with aches and pains.

Once you can run forty-five minutes without stopping, you will easily be able to run an entire 5K. Run your 5K between 75 percent and 85 percent of your maximum heart rate and *enjoy* your run.

CYCLING

Cycling is another great exercise, and it can be used as an alternative or complement to running. Cycling came to my attention in 2005, the year I was competing for *The Biggest Loser* prize. Lance Armstrong made the news that summer because he was competing in the Tour de France. Lance Armstrong was a huge motivation for me during my own weight loss competition. Remember in Chapter 4 I talked about teammates? Well, Lance never knew it, but I considered him a *virtual* teammate.

I can remember in the evenings after a long workout, I would be tired and I would sit down to watch the Tour de France on TV. The network would go in-depth about the training habits of these cyclists and of Lance Armstrong in particular. I learned that the majority of the training that Lance did was in his aerobic range. Of course there were a couple of exceptions—when he was doing the time trials and when he was in the mountains. At those times, he was absolutely up in his anaerobic range. And of course near the end of any stage, he would get up into his actual VO_2 max as he sprinted toward the finish line. But the majority of the work that Lance did was in his aerobic range.

That knowledge helped me understand that even when I was cycling, I needed to ensure that I kept a very good fairly fast pace. At that time, I started to ride my bicycle to and from the gym. I made sure that I kept my heart rate near the upper end of my aerobic range. I would not just coast along at an easy pace. I would actually work hard on the way to the gym, even though the cycling was not my primary workout.

One of my students in 2008 lost 44 pounds in one summer through cycling. He had bad knees, so over eight weeks during the summer he rode the recumbent bike in his living room. He worked out both in his aerobic range and in his anaerobic range. He used interval training, as I've discussed in a previous chapter, and lost 44 pounds. So you absolutely can do this on a bike; you just have to pay attention to your heart rate.

When you're cycling for weight loss, you must keep these things in mind:

- Keep constant pressure on the pedals—no coasting.
- Focus on your heart rate. I wear my heart rate monitor whenever I get on the bike. If you want to get fancier you can buy bike-mounted computers that track your pace, your heart rate, and lots of other stuff. I just focus on keeping my heart rate within my aerobic range at a minimum, so I keep it simple.
- Hit the hills hard. Whenever I come to a hill I determine that I'm going to "kill the hills." In other words, I'm going to hit the hill hard and go up as fast as I possibly can. I'm not going to climb slowly and I'm not going to get off and walk. This turns any workout into an interval.
- Never, ever coast. On your way down the hill, don't just coast. Return back to your aerobic range. That's when we're cycling for weight loss. You can make a cycling workout very, very effective if you avoid coasting.

SWIMMING FOR WEIGHT LOSS

Swimming is an odd exercise. And I don't just say that because I almost drowned in the San Francisco Bay during my first triathlon. Swimming is unique in that when you become good, it will be hard for you to get an effective workout. Water will support your body so that you can exercise in it, but that buoyancy will also make it difficult to lose pounds.

As you get better in the water, you become more efficient and more fluid. You're inevitably going to cover any distance with less effort. Once you become good at, say, the freestyle stroke, you will move through the water so easily that you will seemingly glide on top of the water and you may barely increase your heart rate. I remember reading the story of the gentleman who swam across the English Channel at just 65 percent of his maximum heart rate. He was overweight, but he was a very efficient swimmer. This efficiency actually makes swimming a great rest day or nonimpact exercise, but not the greatest weight loss exercise.

So if you're going to swim for weight loss, remember to focus on stroke type, speed, and time. You'll either want to cover a lap in as short an amount of time as possible and then get better each session, or you will want to swim for very long periods of time.

Another interesting thing about swimming is that it may promote the retention of an extra layer of fat. I recently read a study that found female college swimmers had slightly higher body fat percentages than their non-swimming athletic counterparts. It was surmised that maybe the body knows that it is more efficient with an extra layer of fat, so the body retains this extra layer for performance. Of course there is an exception to everything, and Olympic medalist Dara Torres is one of those exceptions who regularly displays her incredibly fit physique. It is also interesting to note that she swims short, very fast distances, which even in swimming are called sprints.

Again, when it comes to losing it forever through swimming alone, your weight loss swimming is going to be time-based unless you swim harder strokes. If you're swimming the butterfly stroke, then you may be able to put in less time because your effort is going to be more intense. But if you're doing the freestyle or the breaststroke, you're going to have to put a lot of time in the water to make it effective for weight loss.

STAY MOTIVATED

Remember that whichever exercises you choose to supplement your ABC Circuits, try to become an "–er." What I mean is, don't just run, become a runner. Don't just bike, become a biker. Don't just swim, become a swimmer. Learn all the ins and outs of the activity you plan to pursue and invest your time and money into that activity. Learning and investing in the activity is necessary if you're going to enjoy the activity, which will be essential if you're going to lose those pounds forever and reach your long-term goal.

I do quite a bit of motivational speaking around the country, and people have told me that they find my running quote helps motivate them when they want to quit:

Running is a metaphor for life. We're all runners. We're either running away from something or running toward something. On days when I have no motivation I lace up my shoes and do it anyway. On those days I'm running from the old Pete. On days that I feel good I'm running toward something: I'm running toward my future. The key for me is that no matter what, when the sun comes up, I'd better be running.

KEY POINTS

- Running strengthens the heart and lungs and lowers negative health risk factors.
- The focus is on your heart rate and time, not on speed and distance.
- When you're cycling for weight loss, you need to:
  - Keep constant pressure on the pedals—no coasting
  - Focus on your heart rate
  - Hit the hills hard
- Losing it forever through swimming is going to be time-based unless you swim harder strokes.

CHAPTER 14 CHALLENGES

New Challenges | Run Twice a Week for the Next Few Weeks

If you haven't tried running yet, try running twice a week for thirty to sixty minutes. Pick somewhere pleasant to run if you can so you can enjoy the outdoors. If you already run a little bit, complete a run that is an hour and a half within your aerobic range. If you want further guidance, check out the running plan in this chapter.

Find a Class

Find a beginners' running class that focuses on heart rate training in order to learn how to maximize your running.

Ongoing Challenges | Check with Your Physician Before Running

If you haven't had a physical with your physician yet, schedule one so that you can start running, biking, or swimming on your noncircuit days.

Stretch

Make sure you do the stretches I've outlined before you do any exercise, especially running.

Weigh In

Time to weigh yourself, as you should be doing every week. Did you reach your goal of losing that Forever Five? Make sure you celebrate by commenting at www.PeteThomas.com and trumpet your success!

FOREVER FUNDAMENTALS—
STEP TWO CHECKLIST

NOW THAT WE'VE GONE THROUGH STEP 2: YOUR PLAN, WE SHOULD BE making even more small, incremental—and permanent—changes. Remember this is about life change, so each Forever Habit we incorporate into our lives should be celebrated. Whether we lose a pound a week or a month, we want that weight to never, ever come back. You should have formed, or be in the process of forming, the following Forever Habits as you seek to truly Manage Your Mouth and Multiply Your Muscles. Make note of the habits that you need to work on and try and come up with a plan to start implementing them.

STEP 2: YOUR PLAN FOREVER HABITS

- Think of food as fuel, not as a reward.
- Write down daily calories in your LIF2 Success Journal.
- Eat within your Personal Daily Fuel Goal (first you have to figure it out).
- Make small modifications to your food to reduce calories.
- Keep your cupboards clear of bad or trigger foods.
- Figure out your macronutrient ratio and stick to it.
- Keep in mind Correct Calories, Cautious Carbs for every meal.
- Avoid the white poisons—sugar, salt, and refined flour.
- Keep blood sugar stable by eating very few bad carbs.
- Avoid bad carbs at night, when they can block release of HGH.
- Eat a good breakfast within thirty minutes of waking up.
- Eat a thoughtful evening meal that doesn't load up on calories or carbs.
- Don't eat in front of the TV.
- Have Three Fs with every meal: fluid, filler, feast.
- Deliberate grocery shopping: "If it's not on the list, I must resist".
- Form new nutrition habits, such as drinking water instead of soda and dipping salad bites in salad dressing rather than pouring it on.
- Eat according to your Perfect Personalized Forever Meal Plan.
- Plan what you're going to eat at a restaurant or party before you go.
- Plan regular exercise into your schedule, whenever the best time is.
- Communicate regularly with your team as you work out, including your medical team before you begin.
- Exercise intensely, based on heart rate.
- Exercise according to your Perfect Personalized Forever Workout Plan, using the F.I.T.T. principle to determine Frequency, Intensity, Time, and Type.
- Warm up with easy cardio and dynamic stretching before every workout.
- Cool down with static stretching after every workout.
- Drink plenty of water (ideally half your body weight in ounces).
- Record workouts in your LIF2 Success Journal.
- Maintain an "active" rest day.

- Maintain a healthy running habit based on staying within your aerobic range.
- Always work out in proper shoes.

AND NOW, A WORD FROM YOUR SPONSOR

Following these principles has made me the weight loss success I am today, more than seven years after leaving *The Biggest Loser*. If you feel like you want to skip one or more of these habits, feel free to move on to another. However, if you find the scale is not moving as you would expect, I can assure you from years of experience helping others that the reason lies in the fact that you are missing one of the components listed here, however small it may appear. Whenever my weight has fluctuated by even a couple of pounds, I have gone back and reviewed the principles I have slacked off on implementing. In other words, I go back to the basics.

MOVING ON

Once we have implemented the principles from this step, we are ready for the next leg in the journey. In Step 3: Your Pursuit, we build on the Forever Habits we've formed but begin to apply them more aggressively so we can Lose It Fast.

STEP THREE
YOUR PURSUIT

"All out it was hard. I did things that I have never done before and coach [Pete Thomas] pushed me above and beyond my limits that I never thought I could do . . . I loved the push, the people, the drive to get to my goals. I still have a long way to go, but my horizon is looking bright and I am on my way to a better life, full circle."

—LISA, LIF2 STUDENT

CHAPTER

THINK FAST

"HEY, PETE, NBC IS GIVING AWAY A $100,000 PRIZE TO THE CONTESTANT who loses the most weight at home."

I told you before that I was voted off *The Biggest Loser* Ranch after sixty-two days. I had been home for four months and had already hit my goal weight. But now—forty-five days before the finale—the network had announced the at-home goal. I had already gotten my health together; now I had the opportunity to maximize my efforts and take home a prize.

I thought to myself, "Wow, that is amazing! If I lose the most weight at home, I could win a $100,000 prize." So I took my workouts to a new level, from two and a half hours a day back up to three and a half or four hours a day.

I worked out five days a week with two off days and ate 2500 calories a day. The two days that I took off were Sunday and Wednesday. Let me tell you about the last workout I did before each off day.

This was the last hour of the last day I would work out before my off day. I called it my Fourth Hour Killer Workout. If you know anything about Jillian Michaels, my trainer on *The Biggest Loser*, you will not be surprised when I tell you that I got this workout from her. I turned on the treadmill, put the incline on 12, put the speed on 10, and then hopped on the treadmill and sprinted for two minutes straight. Have you ever tried sprinting uphill for two whole minutes? It's exhausting! After that I stood on the side for a minute to try to recover, then hopped back on the treadmill and sprinted for two minutes, then stood panting on the side for another minute. I repeated that for one hour straight, and then I fell off the treadmill and prayed that somebody would call the ambulance because I thought I was about to pass out and die.

That is a killer workout. Somebody asked me recently, "Pete, do you ever do that workout now?" Of course, being the confident manly man that I am, I poked my chest out and my ego bubbled to the surface as I considered the silliness of such a question. Then I thought about it and stated with a whimper, "No. That's what you do when there's money on the line."

TIME TO PURSUE IT

I know you've been focused on losing it forever by developing new Forever Habits. I commend you and I'm proud of you. But now it's time to sharpen your focus and not let distractions keep you from eating and exercising properly in this next step.

By now, you should be regularly applying all the principles you've learned and you are well on your way to creating a new lifestyle based on Forever Habits. You have a team around you and proper goals to keep you focused. You know how to reward yourself and have experienced the joy of eating within your Personal Daily Fuel Goal in every environment, including holidays. You should have developed a Personalized Meal Plan with modified foods for an entire month and a personal grocery list that keeps you from straying from that plan.

By now you may even be exercising six days a week according to your Personal Weekly Workouts with a variety of cardio and resistance workouts, including some fat-burning ABC Circuits. You should be working out within or above your aerobic range so that you can maximize your time in the gym. You should be writing in your LIF2 Success Journal and keeping track of your exercise so you can see your progression. You are celebrating every new lifestyle Forever Habit change and pounds lost by touching a teammate on the website.

In a nutshell, you've learned how to Master Your Mind, Manage Your Mouth, and Multiply Your Muscles. You already may be losing a bunch of weight, but now you're ready to push it up a level. Maybe you want to get ready for that special event and you need a little extra push and a little extra challenge. You've come to the right section. Welcome to Lose It Fast.

As I've explained, for me that special event was my *Biggest Loser* live finale at the end of November 2005. I had already reached my goal weight, but I wanted to get rid of another 35 or so pounds in order to win the $100,000 At-Home Prize. I still did it by applying my Forever Habits until I lost that next pound, but I applied them in a more aggressive, stricter fashion. I was able to do that because I had already created a "new me" over the summer. And now I was ready to rely on and apply everything I had learned up to that point to Lose It Fast.

NEW GUIDELINES FOR EATING OUT

You've got to be really mindful of how you eat during this step. Ideally you will eat out less and eat your own food more than you have been, but there are times when you are either traveling or a situation comes up that forces you to eat at a restaurant. Don't give in to temptation; stay strong. Here are some pointers for eating out in this step.

- Don't eat at a restaurant unless you've looked up the calorie contents online.
- Choose what you'll eat before you step inside the restaurant and stick with it.
- Take your scale with you and only eat foods you can measure.

I'm sure you know this program well enough by now that you can come up with your own guidelines for eating out during Step 3: Your Pursuit. The LIF2 community needs to hear them, so come and share them at www.PeteThomas.com.

CARDIO COCKTAIL

Up to this point, I have not really introduced two-a-day workouts or similar concepts. Now, before you get turned off, I don't want you to think two-a-day workouts are just for football players. Actually, you would be surprised at how many amateur triathletes and goal-oriented people just like you work out multiple times a day. They just find a way to squeeze it in. And so will you.

I want to mention a simple concept called the cardio cocktail. Every evening right before bed, I would do a really hard thirty-minute run at 85 percent of my aerobic maximum or above. My warm-up would be minimal, because I would hop on the treadmill and just start pushing it from the very first minute. Obviously I do not recommend this as a regular practice; I am just giving an example. I would complete this hard run and be so tired that all I could do was shower, drink some water, and hit the bed. Hard workouts like this one are the type of workouts you do when your goal is within sight.

To help you reach Your Pursuit goal, I've included twelve weeks of secondary workouts following my Lose It Fast 12-Week Workout Plan in Chapter 17.

MORE TIME

As my story illustrates, if you want improved results, you've got to increase a couple of variables in our F.I.T.T. equation. In this case, I increased my time from two and a half hours to four hours a day. I also increased my intensity to get over the plateau I had experienced.

I wish I could tell you there was a magic food or pill that would take out this "sweat" element, but the truth is, the miracle starts with your getting into the gym and putting in some more time and effort. Then the miracle of 1 pound a week will turn into the miracle of 1 pound every three days, or in my case a little over 1 pound every single day. It's hard work, but that's when the results really get amazing.

So are you ready to roll up your sleeves and get to work? I mean really work? If so, let's go.

"I wanted to be able to walk upstairs without being out of breath. I wanted to be healthier, I wanted to be more active, I didn't want to be the kind of person who sits on the couch all the time. I wanted to feel better about myself. So after I lost 40 pounds, I went shopping with the girls in the beginning of September and bought new clothes, because pretty much none of my dress clothes from last year fit."

—ELLEN, LIF2 STUDENT

CHAPTER

16

LOSE IT FAST GOALS

HOPEFULLY YOU'VE BEEN REWARDING YOURSELF FOR EVERY NEW Forever Habit and every Forever Five pounds lost with a non-food treat or some fitness-related purchase. You might want to think of more compelling rewards for this step. Maybe a special trip to the spa or a deep tissue massage or a night away with that special someone. A nice concrete reward is going to make those "high" portions of your H.I.I.T. intervals a little more bearable. As you're trying to sprint on the treadmill at an incline of 13, keep those gifts to yourself in the front of your mind.

Maybe it's time to purchase a new dress or suit that you'll be able to fit into when you reach your Pursuit goal weight. Hang it where you can see it. When you reach your goal, you will parade around in that outfit like you are half of the royal couple. I told you in an earlier chapter that the prospect of fitting into that sweet white suit kept me motivated during many a long workout on the ranch.

Or maybe an event itself is the payoff. If you're going to be attending a friend's wedding or taking a vacation in a tropical location and want to look amazing, then attending the actual event will be your reward.

You get the idea. Your rewards should intensify along with your work in this step.

SHARPER FOCUS

Maybe in the past few weeks you've had a day or two a week when your calories inched up over your Personal Daily Fuel Goal, and you just made up for it the following day. No more of that in this step. What you'll need in this step is 90 percent compliance 100 percent of the time. Do you have the focus for that? You will if you continually focus on that next workout and the next day. Review your Personal Success Statement as well as your Personal Power Goals every day to keep your head in the game. I will ask you to rewrite them in just a few pages.

LOSE IT FAST—TEAMMATES

You must already have a team in place to fully succeed in this step of the journey. You should have let go of the negative people in your life a while ago. Over the next few weeks, you will need people who totally believe in you and your ability to do amazing things. And you may need to add another member to the team.

Let me put it plainly. You need a drill sergeant on your team. I strongly suggest you get a trainer for this step of your weight loss. Be careful, however, because trainers come in all shapes and sizes and range from good, better, to best. Many trainers know how to use the machines at the gym, but they don't necessarily know much about metabolic training, running at the upper end of your aerobic range, and other fat-burning secrets. A great trainer will help you achieve your goals in the gym without allowing you to slack. They will keep you focused and teach you to use new equipment and techniques without hurting yourself. And, sad to say, good ones are hard to come by. You need someone who will call it like it is, demand the best of you, and push you to the finish line.

And remember, this step is not forever. You will reach your goal and then move into maintenance and focus on your life's purpose.

YOU MAY NEED TO SHUFFLE YOUR TEAM

One of the ways that reality shows provide a fresh twist is to shuffle teams. On my season of *The Biggest Loser,* the men's team kept beating the women week after week because the women were caught up in fighting instead of protecting their best competitors. So the producers came up with the idea of dividing us into smaller teams of two.

And guess who got to choose the teams? You got it, yours truly. After thinking and praying about it, I finally made the decision that the teams would be based on who would work best together in losing massive amounts of weight. I paired myself with the most encouraging guy on the ranch, Dr. Jeff, who physically was not the strongest contestant on the ranch.

This matchup got me voted off in the very next episode. I could have easily chosen Matt, who was destined to have a huge week on the scale. But I'm still glad I did it because Dr. Jeff was a great encouragement to me, and our friendship has endured. The other contestants all went on to lose a lot of weight, at least in part because they got strong competitors as new teammates.

You might need a fresh new team for this new step. The next few weeks are going to be very intense, physically and emotionally. Is there someone you know who works out a little harder than you, maybe a person who is more advanced in her workouts? You might want to enlist her as a workout partner to push you.

Is there a super-positive person around you who always sees the bright side of things? They might be willing to join your team and help you see the bright side when you're not seeing that next pound drop off as fast as you'd like. The corollary to this is that you may have to terminate some negative people from your team. I don't mean terminate as in TV mafia terminations; I mean you gently let them go from your inner circle. Negative people will greatly hinder you in this stage. I recommend you come over to www.PeteThomas.com and find online teammates to help keep you focused. Read the stories of others who have entered the Pursuit step to keep yourself motivated.

CHALLENGE YOURSELF TO 100 PERCENT COMPLIANCE

You really have to Manage Your Mouth in this step. No more slipping in extra calories above your Personal Daily Fuel Goal and making up for it the next day. No more spontaneous, "Hey, this looks good, let me eat it and reduce my calories tonight."

No, for the next few weeks you'll be on one of those set plans I described in an earlier chapter. What I mean is that I will give you a new Personal Daily Fuel Goal and you'll have to create a menu that falls within that Personal Daily Fuel Goal range. Don't feel like creating another menu? Fine, you can use mine. It's a set plan, but you are welcome to create your own set plan, and I will give you some guidelines for doing so.

One of the reasons the Lose It Forever steps work so well is that they are flexible enough to fit into any lifestyle. But the Pursuit step is not about flexibility, it's about sticking to your nutrition and exercise plan so that you can Lose It Fast. I still want you to concentrate on your Forever Habits, but you'll have to be stricter with your mouth than you have been up to this point. Let me give you some guidelines to help you create your set plan for this step's food plan.

LOSE THE WHITE POISONS

We can reach our goals faster if we lose the white poisons—sugar, salt, and refined flour—that I talked about in Chapter 7 from our diets. This is difficult if you consume a lot of processed food. Processed food contains a lot of sugar to add flavor, so be careful of that. Avoiding sugar is going to be key to losing weight at this stage.

As I said before, salt is a weight loss killer. And fried food will be a no-no during this time. The body considers flour a carbohydrate, so there's going to be an insulin response when that happens, followed by a perceptible energy crash. That can lead to an even stronger white poison craving, so let's work hard to avoid the white poisons as much as possible in this step.

CHOOSE YOUR FOOD WEAPONS

There are certain foods that were a *must* for me during my Pursuit step. These foods were regular staples of my food plan and I included them in nearly every meal. They included lean proteins, fats, and fresh vegetables.

MORE WATER

My normal recommendation is to drink one half of your body weight in ounces a day. That means if you weigh 150 pounds, you should already be consuming 75 ounces of water a day. Now you're going to add a little more. Men will drink approximately 1 gallon, or 128 ounces, and ladies will drink approximately 100 ounces. And as much as possible, we want to switch to drinking distilled water.

This extra water will help suppress your appetite so you don't get hunger cravings throughout the day. Water also increases your body's ability to metabolize fat, so we don't want to neglect that either.

When it comes to water, the best thing that you can do is to drink water that is very, very cold. If you drink ice-cold water, the body has to bring that up to your body's internal temperature. The body burns extra calories simply to bring ice-cold water up to the temperature of the body. This caloric burn is minimal, but every little bit helps!

SECRET WEAPON—CALORIC CYCLING

When it comes to caloric cycling, you can adjust the number of calories that you take in a day to keep the body guessing as to what's coming. I explained caloric cycling in Chapter 5. Well, it's time to implement it now.

Following this regimen will accomplish a couple of things in your diet journey. One, you will have a little more food on the weekends, which will help you emotionally. Two, you will keep the body guessing because it doesn't know exactly how many calories are coming. It's an advanced concept, and it's time to use it as we Lose It Fast.

STEP IT UP—LOSE IT FAST AND FASTER

This step is going to require that you redouble your exercise efforts. You will have to really focus and Multiply Your Muscles with renewed intensity if you're going to Lose It Fast. That's a good thing, because if you've been cruising along with your own exercise program for a period of time, your body may have adapted to the exercise you've been doing.

In fact, you may have hit a plateau where you haven't seen the scale move much. So it's time to step it up and increase the intensity of your workouts so that you can get that scale to move again in the right direction. Now it's time for you to use your Personalized Lose It Fast Workout Plan. But first, let's start with some guidelines to help you develop your own Pursuit step workouts.

H.I.I.T. IT

If you're following my guidelines, you're already doing cardio twice a week, on Wednesday and Saturday. Most people choose to do steady state on those days, which is fine as you Lose It Forever. For Lose It Fast, I want you to transform that steady state into high-intensity interval training.

In other words, you're going to alternate between high-intensity and low-intensity intervals the entire time you're working out. And you're not going to stop to rest between the intervals. You can get some ideas and sample workouts from Chapter 11.

Previously I talked about working within our aerobic range, which is 75 to 85 percent of our maximum heart rate. To really Lose It Fast, we need to be working at the top of this range throughout our workouts now. Try to stay around 85 percent of your max, or even a little higher during the intense portions of the H.I.I.T.

RESISTANCE X 4

In Chapter 12, I introduced some powerful fat-burning exercises called the ABCs of High-Intensity Circuit Resistance Training. I know from experience that most people will not want to stick with intense circuit training programs forever.

But if you really want to Lose It Fast, you're going to have to do your best circuits. Which means following the workouts in this step and being strict about doing your resistance workouts all four times during the week. You're still only working each muscle twice with two days of rest in between, but you're working much harder and spending more time exercising. Combine that with the H.I.I.T. workouts on Wednesday and Saturday and watch the pounds come off.

CHAPTER 16 CHALLENGES

New Challenges | H.I.I.T. Twice a Week

We're going to replace our steady state cardio on Wednesday and Saturday with high-intensity interval training. Remember to stay at the top of your aerobic range, 85 percent or higher of your max heart rate. If you need a reminder about this, reread Chapter 11.

Do Circuits X 4

Increase your resistance circuits to four times a week. Do the circuits in the Lose It Fast 12-Week Workout Plan in Chapter 17. They not only alternate push and pull muscles but also work out the larger muscles first to maximize efficiency.

Lose It Fast Plan

Fill in the blanks below and follow the associated instructions for the next twelve weeks.

MASTER YOUR MIND

My Personal Success Statement (recite twice daily)

_____

_____

_____
_____

My Personal Power Goals, aka My Top 3 Lose It Fast Goals (recite twice daily)

_____
_____
_____
_____

Touch a teammate today and update him or her on my accomplishment (in person, by phone, text, social media website)

MANAGE YOUR MOUTH
Personal Daily Fuel Goal

Women	1200 to 1400 calories
Men	1600 to 1800 calories

Track your calories daily and maintain them within this range for the next twelve weeks.

Personal daily water intake   100 to 128 ounces

"Lose It Fast, Lose It Forever has been easy to understand and work with. I like the emphasis on modification of the everyday foods that I eat. I have three kids who are all into sports and we are always on the go, so fast food has been a main staple in our diets. The program has taught me to change what we eat. As of today I have lost 105 pounds!"

—KEITH, LIF2 STUDENT

"I said to Pete, 'What is it that I need to do to lose this weight? I'm not looking to take three years to do this. I want to do this as quickly as possible.' He said, 'No problem; how much time can you give me in the gym?' I started doing those exercises right away and the weight just started coming off. Of course, once I started losing weight, that really made me more excited. It's been so rewarding. I weigh less now than I did when I was sixteen."

—CHRIS, LIF2 STUDENT

CHAPTER

17

YOUR PERSONALIZED PURSUIT MEAL AND WORKOUT PLANS

PERSONALIZED MEAL PLAN

WHEN I AM in the Pursuit phase, the foods I include in my weekly menu are similar to the ones I included in Chapter 8, so I will not include a sample menu here. If you don't want to create your own meal plan, feel free to use the one I included before. However, be aware that my portion sizes will change a little bit because I will reduce my Personal Daily Fuel Goal to help me lose those Forever Five, or however many I'm shooting for. As a reminder, we learned how to calculate our current and goal weight in Chapter 5. Once you decide on a goal weight for Your Pursuit phase, go to www.PeteThomas.com and you will find a calculator to determine your new Personal Daily Fuel Goal.

Once I have created my own Personalized Pursuit Meal Plan, I follow that plan for the next twelve weeks. It becomes, in essence, a set plan. Once you create your own plan, you should follow it religiously as well.

Although I include some variety in my Pursuit Meal Plan, my calorie percentages per meal will be consistent. For instance, I usually consume around 20 percent of the calories in my Personal Daily Fuel Goal at breakfast, 30 percent of my daily calories at lunch, 40 percent at dinner, and around 10 percent as snacks throughout the day.

This plan is designed for variety and discipline. So rather than eating what's in my plan, I would like you to create your own Pursuit Meal Plan to fit your goals and life circumstances. You have to personalize it in order to ensure your own compliance! Select veggies, snacks, fruit, and condiments from Chapter 8. Remember to avoid extra salt, carbohydrates, and refined flour foods. Blank Personalized Lose It Fast set meal plan forms are available at www.PeteThomas.com. Or fill out a form like the one below—the same one you used when you created your Perfect Personalized Forever Meal Plan.

MY WEEKLY PURSUIT MEAL PLAN—BREAKFAST (LUNCH/DINNER)

	Fluid	Filler	Feast
Sunday			
Monday			
Tuesday			
Wednesday			
Thursday			
Friday			
Saturday			

PERSONALIZED WORKOUT PLAN

Fill in the blanks below and memorize your numbers, then follow the workouts below for the next twelve weeks. Begin with the warm-up stretches and end with the cooldown stretches.

Multiply Your Muscles

My aerobic heart rate range is _____ to _____ beats per minute.

Your goal is to average 85 percent of maximum and above for the duration of your workouts. As a reminder, for women, your maximum heart rate is 220 minus your age. For men, your maximum heart rate is 226 minus your age.

PETE THOMAS'S STANDARD WARM-UP AND COOLDOWN STRETCHES

These warm-ups and cooldowns are explained in more detail in Chapter 11.

Warm-up Stretches

- Light Jogging (75% HR)
- Side Shuffles
- Carioca with Twists
- High Knee Skips
- Butt Kicks
- Knee Hug Walk

Cooldown Stretches

- Half Neck Rolls to the Front and Back
- Standing Quad Stretch
- Butterfly (inner thighs, groin, hips, lower back)
- Hamstring/Back Stretch
- Seated IT Band
- Lower Back Stretch

PETE THOMAS'S LOSE IT FAST 12-WEEK WORKOUT PLAN

You will find descriptions of all of these exercises following the workout plan.

Note: When doing ABC Circuits, perform each exercise for one minute, then move to the next exercise in order. After you complete all three exercises in order (one circuit), start over until you complete the circuit three times. Then move to the next circuit with as little rest as possible in between circuits.

LOSE IT FAST WORKOUT—WEEK 1

	Circuit 1	Circuit 2	Circuit 3	Circuit 4	Circuit 5	Cardio Circuit
MONDAY—PUSH	**A** Modified Push-ups from Knees **B** Wall Sits **C** Jumping Jacks	**A** DB Chest Presses **B** Air Squats **C** Butt Kickers	**A** Dumbbell Shoulder Presses **B** Sumo Squats **C** Fast Feet	**A** Overhead Triceps Presses—right arm **C** Jumping Jacks **B** Sit-ups	**A** Overhead Triceps Press—left arm **C** Butt Kickers **B** Crunches	**C** Fast Feet **C** Jumping Jacks **C** Butt Kickers
TUESDAY—PULL	**A** One Arm Row—right arm **B** Pelvic Thrusts **C** Ice Skaters with Hop	**A** One Arm Row—left arm **B** Reverse Lunges **C** Jog in Place	**A** Supermans **B** Forward Lunges **C** Jump Rope in Place	**A** Biceps Curls—right arm **C** Ice Skaters with Hop **B** Bicycles	**A** Biceps Curls—left arm **C** Jog in Place **B** Side Heel Touches	**C** Jump Rope in Place **C** Ice Skaters with Hop **C** Jog in Place
WEDNESDAY	1- Hour Cardio H.I.I.T. or SS (LSD)					
THURSDAY—PUSH	**A** Modified Push-ups from Knees **B** Wall Sits **C** Jumping Jacks	**A** DB Chest Press **B** Air Squats **C** Butt Kickers	**A** Dumbbell Shoulder Press **B** Sumo Squat **C** Fast Feet	**A** Overhead Triceps Presses—right arm **C** Jumping Jacks **B** Sit-ups	**A** Overhead Triceps Press—left arm **C** Butt Kickers **B** Crunches	**C** Fast Feet **C** Jumping Jacks **C** Butt Kickers
FRIDAY—PULL	**A** One Arm Row—right arm **B** Pelvic Thrusts **C** Ice Skaters with Hop	**A** One Arm Row—left arm **B** Reverse Lunges **C** Jog in Place	**A** Supermans **B** Forward Lunges **C** Jump Rope in Place	**A** Biceps Curls—right arm **C** Ice Skaters with Hop **B** Bicycles	**A** Biceps Curls—left arm **C** Jog in Place **B** Side Heel Touches	**C** Jump Rope in Place **C** Ice Skaters with Hop **C** Jog in Place
SATURDAY	1-Hour Cardio H.I.I.T. or SS (LSD)					
SUNDAY	Active Rest Day					

Pete Thomas's Lose It Fast 12-Week Workout Plan

LOSE IT FAST WORKOUT—WEEK 2

	Circuit 1	Circuit 2	Circuit 3	Circuit 4	Circuit 5	Cardio Circuit
MONDAY—PUSH	**A** Modified Push-ups from Knees **B** Wall Sits **C** Jumping Jacks	**A** DB Chest Presses **B** Air Squats **C** Butt Kickers	**A** Dumbbell Shoulder Presses **B** Sumo Squats **C** Fast Feet	**A** Overhead Tricep Presses—right arm **C** Jumping Jacks **B** Sit-ups	**A** Overhead Tricep Presses—left arm **C** Butt Kickers **B** Crunches	**C** Fast Feet **C** Jumping Jacks **C** Butt Kickers
TUESDAY—PULL	**A** One Arm Row—right arm **B** Pelvic Thrusts **C** Ice Skaters with Hop	**A** One Arm Row—left arm **B** Reverse Lunges **C** Jog in Place	**A** Supermans **B** Forward Lunges **C** Jump Rope in Place	**A** Biceps Curls—right arm **C** Ice Skaters with Hop **B** Bicycles	**A** Biceps Curls—left arm **C** Jog in Place **B** Side Heel Touches	**C** Jump Rope in Place **C** Ice Skaters with Hop **C** Jog in Place
WEDNESDAY	1-Hour Cardio H.I.I.T. or SS (LSD)					
THURSDAY—PUSH	**A** Modified Push-ups from Knees **B** Wall Sits **C** Jumping Jacks	**A** DB Chest Presses **B** Air Squats **C** Butt Kickers	**A** Dumbbell Shoulder Presses **B** Sumo Squats **C** Fast Feet	**A** Overhead Triceps Presses—right arm **C** Jumping Jacks **B** Sit-ups	**A** Overhead Triceps Presses—left arm **C** Butt Kickers **B** Crunches	**C** Fast Feet **C** Jumping Jacks **C** Butt Kickers
FRIDAY—PULL	**A** One Arm Row—right arm **B** Pelvic Thrusts **C** Ice Skaters with Hop	**A** One Arm Row—left arm **B** Reverse Lunges **C** Jog in Place	**A** Supermans **B** Forward Lunges **C** Jump Rope in Place	**A** Biceps Curls—right arm **C** Ice Skaters with Hop **B** Bicycles	**A** Biceps Curls—left arm **C** Jog in Place **B** Side Heel Touches	**C** Jump Rope in Place **C** Ice Skaters with Hop **C** Jog in Place
SATURDAY	1-Hour Cardio H.I.I.T. or SS (LSD)					
SUNDAY	Active Rest Day					

Pete Thomas's Lose It Fast 12-Week Workout Plan

LOSE IT FAST WORKOUT—WEEK 3

	Circuit 1	Circuit 2	Circuit 3	Circuit 4	Circuit 5	Cardio Circuit
MONDAY—PUSH	**A** Standard Push-ups **B** Prisoner Squats **C** Jumping Jacks	**A** DB Chest Flys **B** Side to Side Squats **C** High Knees	**A** Anterior DB Raises **B** Squat Holds **C** 1-2-3 Heismans	**A** Triceps Kick Backs—right arm **C** Jumping Jacks **B** Weighted Sit-ups DB on chest	**A** Triceps Kick Backs—left arm **C** High Knees **B** Raised Knee Crunches	**C** 1-2-3 Heismans **C** Jumping Jacks **C** High Knees
TUESDAY—PULL	**A** DB High Rows (overhand) **B** Side Lunges **C** Side to Side Hops	**A** DB Low Rows (underhand) **B** Static Lunges **C** High Knees	**A** Heavy DB Dead Lifts **B** Traveling Forward Lunges **C** Jog in Place	**A** Concentration Curls—right arm **C** Side to Side Hops **B** Side Rows (legs raised)	**A** Concentration Curls—left arm **C** High Knees **B** Side Bends	**C** Jog in Place **C** Side to Side Hops **C** High Knees
WEDNESDAY	1-Hour Cardio H.I.I.T. or SS (LSD)					
THURSDAY—PUSH	**A** Standard Push-ups **B** Prisoner Squats **C** Jumping Jacks	**A** DB Chest Flys **B** Side to Side Squats **C** High Knees	**A** Anterior DB Raise **B** Squat Holds **C** 1-2-3 Heismans	**A** Triceps Kick Backs—right arm **C** Jumping Jacks **B** Weighted Sit-ups DB on chest	**A** Triceps Kick Backs—left arm **C** High Knees **B** Raised Knee Crunches	**C** 1-2-3 Heismans **C** Jumping Jacks **C** High Knees
FRIDAY—PULL	**A** DB High Rows (overhand) **B** Side Lunges **C** Side to Side Hops	**A** DB Low Rows (underhand) **B** Static Lunges **C** High Knees	**A** Heavy DB Dead Lifts **B** Traveling Forward Lunges **C** Jog in Place	**A** Concentration Curls—right arm **C** Side to Side Hops **B** Side Rows (legs raised)	**A** Concentration Curls—left arm **C** High Knees **B** Side Bends	**C** Jog in Place **C** Side to Side Hops **C** High Knees
SATURDAY	1-Hour Cardio H.I.I.T. or SS (LSD)					
SUNDAY	Active Rest Day					

Pete Thomas's Lose It Fast 12-Week Workout Plan

LOSE IT FAST WORKOUT—WEEK 4

	Circuit 1	Circuit 2	Circuit 3	Circuit 4	Circuit 5	Cardio Circuit
MONDAY—PUSH	**A** Standard Push-ups **B** Prisoner Squats **C** Jumping Jacks	**A** DB Chest Flys **B** Side to Side Squats **C** High Knees	**A** Anterior DB Raises **B** Squat Holds **C** 1-2-3 Heismans	**A** Triceps Kick Backs—right arm **C** Jumping Jacks **B** Weighted Sit-ups DB on chest	**A** Triceps Kick Backs—left arm **C** High Knees **B** Raised Knee Crunches	**C** 1-2-3 Heismans **C** Jumping Jacks **C** High Knees
TUESDAY—PULL	**A** DB High Rows (overhand) **B** Side Lunges **C** Side to Side Hops	**A** DB Low Rows (underhand) **B** Static Lunges **C** High Knees	**A** Heavy DB Dead Lifts **B** Traveling Forward Lunges **C** Jog in Place	**A** Concentration Curl—right arm **C** Side to Side Hops **B** Side Rows (legs raised)	**A** Concentration Curl—left arm **C** High Knees **B** Side Bends	**C** Jog in Place **C** Side to Side Hops **C** High Knees
WEDNESDAY	1-Hour Cardio H.I.I.T. or SS (LSD)					
THURSDAY—PUSH	**A** Standard Push-ups **B** Prisoner Squats **C** Jumping Jacks	**A** DB Chest Flys **B** Side to Side Squats **C** High Knees	**A** Anterior DB Raises **B** Squat Holds **C** 1-2-3 Heismans	**A** Triceps Kick Backs—right arm **C** Jumping Jacks **B** Weighted Sit-ups DB on chest	**A** Triceps Kick Backs—left arm **C** High Knees **B** Raised Knee Crunches	**C** 1-2-3 Heismans **C** Jumping Jacks **C** High Knees
FRIDAY—PULL	**A** DB High Rows (overhand) **B** Side Lunges **C** Side to Side Hops	**A** DB Low Rows (underhand) **B** Static Lunges **C** High Knees	**A** Heavy DB Dead Lifts **B** Traveling Forward Lunges **C** Jog in Place	**A** Concentration Curl—right arm **C** Side to Side Hops **B** Side Rows (legs raised)	**A** Concentration Curl—left arm **C** High Knees **B** Side Bends	**C** Jog in Place **C** Side to Side Hops **C** High Knees
SATURDAY	1-Hour Cardio H.I.I.T. or SS (LSD)					
SUNDAY	Active Rest Day					

Pete Thomas's Lose It Fast 12-Week Workout Plan

LOSE IT FAST WORKOUT—WEEK 5

	Circuit 1	Circuit 2	Circuit 3	Circuit 4	Circuit 5	Cardio Circuit
MONDAY—PUSH	**A** Triangle Push-ups **B** Weighted Sumo Squats **C** Cross-Country Skiers	**A** Heavy DB Chest Presses **B** Squat Hops **C** 5 Count Up Downs	**A** Lateral Raises **B** Squats with a Front Kick **C** Weighted Jumping Jacks	**A** Overhead Triceps Presses—both arms **C** Cross-Country Skiers **B** V Sit-up (knee to chest, rockers)	**A** Triceps Kick Backs—both arms **C** 5 Count Up Downs **B** Plank Hold	**C** Weighted Jumping Jacks **C** Cross-Country Skiers **C** 5 Count Up Downs
TUESDAY—PULL	**A** Bent Over Flys **B** Weighted Forward Lunges **C** Straight Arm Jumping Jacks	**A** Bent Over Y Raise **B** Reverse Lunge to Forward Knee Raise **C** High Knees	**A** Heavy DB Swings **B** Lunge Hold Pulse **C** Cross Arm Jumping Jacks	**A** Hammer Curls **C** Straight Arm Jumping Jacks **B** Side Plank Hold (right)	**A** Biceps Curls (both) **C** High Knees **B** Side Plank Hold (left)	**C** Cross Arm Jumping Jacks **C** Straight Arm Jumping Jacks **C** High Knees
WEDNESDAY	1-Hour Cardio H.I.I.T. or SS (LSD)					
THURSDAY—PUSH	**A** Triangle Push-ups **B** Weighted Sumo Squats **C** Cross-Country Skiers	**A** Heavy DB Chest Presses **B** Squat Hops **C** 5 Count Up Downs	**A** Lateral Raises **B** Squats with a Front Kick **C** Weighted Jumping Jacks	**A** Overhead Triceps Presses—both arms **C** Cross-Country Skiers **B** V Sit-up (knee to chest, rockers)	**A** Triceps Kick Backs—both arms **C** 5 Count Up Downs **B** Plank Hold	**C** Weighted Jumping Jacks **C** Cross Country Skiers **C** 5 Count Up Downs
FRIDAY—PULL	**A** Bent Over Flys **B** Weighted Forward Lunge **C** Straight Arm Jumping Jacks	**A** Bent Over Y Raise **B** Reverse Lunge to Forward Knee Raise **C** High Knees	**A** Heavy DB Swings **B** Lunge Hold Pulse **C** Cross Arm Jumping Jacks	**A** Hammer Curls **C** Straight Arm Jumping Jacks **B** Side Plank Hold (right)	**A** Biceps Curls (both) **C** High Knees **B** Side Plank Hold (left)	**C** Cross Arm Jumping Jacks **C** Straight Arm Jumping Jacks **C** High Knees
SATURDAY	1-Hour Cardio H.I.I.T. or SS (LSD)					
SUNDAY	Active Rest Day					

Pete Thomas's Lose It Fast 12-Week Workout Plan

LOSE IT FAST WORKOUT—WEEK 6

	Circuit 1	Circuit 2	Circuit 3	Circuit 4	Circuit 5	Cardio Circuit
MONDAY—PUSH	**A** Triangle Push-ups **B** Weighted Sumo Squats **C** Cross-Country Skiers	**A** Heavy DB Chest Presses **B** Squat Hops **C** 5 Count Up Downs	**A** Lateral Raises **B** Squats with a Front Kick **C** Weighted Jumping Jacks	**A** Overhead Triceps Presses— both arms **C** Cross-Country Skiers **B** V Sit-ups (knee to chest, rockers)	**A** Triceps Kick Backs— both arms **C** 5 Count Up Downs **B** Plank Hold	**C** Weighted Jumping Jacks **C** Cross Country Skiers **C** 5 Count Up Downs
TUESDAY—PULL	**A** Bent Over Flys **B** Weighted Forward Lunges **C** Straight Arm Jumping Jacks	**A** Bent Over Y Raise **B** Reverse Lunge to Forward Knee Raise **C** High Knees	**A** Heavy DB Swings **B** Lunge Hold Pulse **C** Cross Arm Jumping Jacks	**A** Hammer Curls **C** Straight Arm Jumping Jacks **B** Side Plank Hold (right)	**A** Biceps Curls (both) **C** High Knees **B** Side Plank Hold (left)	**C** Cross Arm Jumping Jacks **C** Straight Arm Jumping Jacks **C** High Knees
WEDNESDAY	1- Hour Cardio H.I.I.T. or SS (LSD)					
THURSDAY—PUSH	**A** Triangle Push-ups **B** Weighted Sumo Squats **C** Cross-Country Skiers	**A** Heavy DB Chest Presses **B** Squat Hops **C** 5 Count Up Downs	**A** Lateral Raises **B** Squats with a Front Kick **C** Weighted Jumping Jacks	**A** Overhead Triceps Presses— both arms **C** Cross-Country Skiers **B** V Sit-up (knee to chest, rockers)	**A** Triceps Kick Backs— both arms **C** 5 Count Up Downs **B** Plank Hold	**C** Weighted Jumping Jacks **C** Cross Country Skiers **C** 5 Count Up Downs
FRIDAY—PULL	**A** Bent Over Flys **B** Weighted Forward Lunges **C** Straight Arm Jumping Jacks	**A** Bent Over Y Raise **B** Reverse Lunge to Forward Knee Raise **C** High Knees	**A** Heavy DB Swings **B** Lunge Hold Pulse **C** Cross Arm Jumping Jacks	**A** Hammer Curls **C** Straight Arm Jumping Jacks **B** Side Plank Hold (right)	**A** Biceps Curls (both) **C** High Knees **B** Side Plank Hold (left)	**C** Cross Arm Jumping Jacks **C** Straight Arm Jumping Jacks **C** High Knees
SATURDAY	1-Hour Cardio H.I.I.T. or SS (LSD)					
SUNDAY	Active Rest Day					

Pete Thomas's Lose It Fast 12-Week Workout Plan

LOSE IT FAST WORKOUT—WEEK 7

	Circuit 1	Circuit 2	Circuit 3	Circuit 4	Circuit 5	Cardio Circuit
MONDAY—PUSH	**A** Explosive Push-ups (from knees) **B** Weighted Squat + Punch **C** Mountain Climbers	**A** DB Pec Decks **B** Deep Sumo Squat—sub 90 degrees (fast) **C** Sumo Jacks	**A** Vertical Rows **B** Jump Squats with Arms Overhead **C** Squat Hops	**A** Triceps Skull Crushers **C** Mountain Climbers **B** Flutter Kicks	**A** Overhead Triceps Press 1 Leg (both arms) **C** Sumo Jacks **B** Scissors	**C** Squat Hops **C** Mountain Climbers **C** Sumo Jacks
TUESDAY—PULL	**A** One Arm DB Snatch (left) **B** Weighted Forward Lunge with Side Twist **C** Plank to Squat	**A** One Arm DB Snatch (right) **B** Reverse Lunge to Forward Knee Raise + Hop **C** Side to Side Donkey Kicks	**A** Weighted Supermans **B** Biceps Curls with Lunges Pulse + Rear Leg Lift **C** 5 Step Floor Touches—Suicides	**A** Reverse Grip Curls **C** Plank to Squat **B** Weighted Cross Body Punching Sit-ups	**A** Biceps Curls (21s) **C** Side to Side Donkey Kicks **B** Side Crunches with Ankle over Knee	**C** 5 Step Floor Touches—Suicides **C** Plank to Squat **C** Side to Side Donkey Kicks
WEDNESDAY	1-Hour Cardio H.I.I.T. or SS (LSD)					
THURSDAY—PUSH	**A** Explosive Push-ups (from knees) **B** Weighted Squat + Punch **C** Mountain Climbers	**A** DB Pec Decks **B** Deep Sumo Squat—sub 90 degrees (fast) **C** Sumo Jacks	**A** Vertical Rows **B** Jump Squats with Arms Overhead **C** Squat Hops	**A** Triceps Skull Crushers **C** Mountain Climbers **B** Flutter Kicks	**A** Overhead Triceps Press 1 Leg (both arms) **C** Sumo Jacks **B** Scissors	**C** Squat Hops **C** Mountain Climbers **C** Sumo Jacks
FRIDAY—PULL	**A** One Arm DB Snatch (left) **B** Weighted Forward Lunge with Side Twist **C** Plank to Squat	**A** One Arm DB Snatch (right) **B** Reverse Lunge to Forward Knee Raise + Hop **C** Side to Side Donkey Kicks	**A** Weighted Supermans **B** Biceps Curls with Lunges Pulse + Rear Leg Lift **C** 5 Step Floor Touches—Suicides	**A** Reverse Grip Curls **C** Plank to Squat **B** Weighted Cross Body Punching Sit-ups	**A** Biceps Curls (21s) **C** Side to Side Donkey Kicks **B** Side Crunches with Ankle over Knee	**C** 5 Step Floor Touches—Suicides **C** Plank to Squat **C** Side to Side Donkey Kicks
SATURDAY	1-Hour Cardio H.I.I.T. or SS (LSD)					
SUNDAY	Active Rest Day					

Pete Thomas's Lose It Fast 12-Week Workout Plan

LOSE IT FAST WORKOUT—WEEK 8

	Circuit 1	Circuit 2	Circuit 3	Circuit 4	Circuit 5	Cardio Circuit
MONDAY—PUSH	**A** Explosive Push-ups (from knees) **B** Weighted Squats + Punch **C** Mountain Climbers	**A** DB Pec Decks **B** Deep Sumo Squats—sub 90 degrees (fast) **C** Sumo Jacks	**A** Vertical Rows **B** Jump Squats with Arms Overhead **C** Squat Hops	**A** Triceps Skull Crushers **C** Mountain Climbers **B** Flutter Kicks	**A** Overhead Triceps Press 1 Leg (both arms) **C** Sumo Jacks **B** Scissors	**C** Squat Hops **C** Mountain Climbers **C** Sumo Jacks
TUESDAY—PULL	**A** One Arm DB Snatches (left) **B** Weighted Forward Lunges with Side Twist **C** Plank to Squat	**A** Onc Arm DB Snatches (right) **B** Reverse Lunge to Forward Knee Raise + Hop **C** Side to Side Donkey Kicks	**A** Weighted Supermans **B** Biceps Curls w Lunges Pulse + Rear Leg Lifts **C** 5 Step Floor Touches— Suicides	**A** Reverse Grip Curls **C** Plank to Squat **B** Weighted Cross Body Punching Sit-ups	**A** Biceps Curls (21s) **C** Side to Side Donkey Kicks **B** Side Crunches with Ankle over Knee	**C** 5 Step Floor Touches— Suicides **C** Plank to Squat **C** Side to Side Donkey Kicks
WEDNESDAY	1-Hour Cardio H.I.I.T. or SS (LSD)					
THURSDAY—PUSH	**A** Explosive Push-ups (from Knees) **B** Weighted Squats + Punch **C** Mountain Climbers	**A** DB Pec Decks **B** Deep Sumo Squats—sub 90 degrees (fast) **C** Sumo Jacks	**A** Vertical Rows **B** Jump Squats with Arms Overhead **C** Squat Hops	**A** Triceps Skull Crushers **C** Mountain Climbers **B** Flutter Kicks	**A** Overhead Triceps Press 1 Leg (both arms) **C** Sumo Jacks **B** Scissors	**C** Squat Hops **C** Mountain Climbers **C** Sumo Jacks
FRIDAY—PULL	**A** One Arm DB Snatches (left) **B** Weighted Forward Lunges with Side Twist **C** Plank to Squat	**A** One Arm DB Snatch (right) **B** Reverse Lunge to Forward Knee Raise + Hop **C** Side to Side Donkey Kicks	**A** Weighted Supermans **B** Biceps Curls with Lunges Pulse + Rear Leg Lifts **C** 5 Step Floor Touches— Suicides	**A** Reverse Grip Curls **C** Plank to Squat **B** Weighted Cross Body Punching Sit-ups	**A** Biceps Curls (21s) **C** Side to Side Donkey Kicks **B** Side Crunches with Ankle over Knee	**C** 5 Step Floor Touches— Suicides **C** Plank to Squat **C** Side to Side Donkey Kicks
SATURDAY	1-Hour Cardio H.I.I.T. or SS (LSD)					
SUNDAY	Active Rest Day					

Pete Thomas's Lose It Fast 12-Week Workout Plan

LOSE IT FAST WORKOUT—WEEK 9

	Circuit 1	Circuit 2	Circuit 3	Circuit 4	Circuit 5	Cardio Circuit
MONDAY—PUSH	**A** Push-ups Rotate to Side Arm Raise **B** Squat Hops (4 Square) **C** Paper Plate Pushes	**A** Heavy DB Chest Flys **B** Squat to Rear Leg Lifts **C** 10 Count Mountain Climber to Squat Hops	**A** Punches with Dumbbells **B** Squat Hold with Skateboarders Kick **C** Burpees	**A** Overhead DB Triceps Press—heavy **C** Paper Plate Pushes **B** Plank to Pointer (opposite arm opposite leg reach)	**A** Alternating Triceps Kick Backs—heavy **C** 10 Count Mountain Climbers to Squat Hops **B** Frog Sit-ups	**C** Burpees **C** Paper Plate Pushes **C** 10 Count Mountain Climbers to Squat Hops
TUESDAY—PULL	**A** Wide Grip Push-ups **B** Single Leg Static Lunges (left leg) **C** High Knee High Arm Sprints in Place	**A** Bent Over Mid-Row (palms in) + Squat Hold **B** Single Leg Static Lunge (right leg) **C** 10 Count Up Down	**A** Single Leg Dead Lifts **B** 3 in 1 Lunge **C** Burpees with Weight	**A** Hammer Curls Heavy (both) **C** High Knee High Arm Sprints in Place **B** Side Plank Dip (left)	**A** Biceps Curls Heavy (both) **C** 10 Count Up Downs **B** Side Plank Dip (right)	**C** Burpees with Weight **C** High Knee High Arm Sprints in Place **C** 10 Count Up Downs
WEDNESDAY	1-Hour Cardio H.I.I.T. or SS (LSD)					
THURSDAY—PUSH	**A** Push-ups Rotate to Side Arm Raises **B** Squat Hops (4 Square) **C** Paper Plate Pushes	**A** Heavy DB Chest Flys **B** Squat to Rear Leg Lifts **C** 10 Count Mountain Climber to Squat Hops	**A** Punches with Dumbbells **B** Squat Hold with Skateboarders Kick **C** Burpees	**A** Overhead DB Triceps Press—Heavy **C** Paper Plate Pushes **B** Plank to Pointer (opposite arm opposite leg reach)	**A** Alternating Triceps Kick Backs—heavy **C** 10 Count Mountain Climbers to Squat Hops **B** Frog Sit-ups	**C** Burpees **C** Paper Plate Pushes **C** 10 Count Mountain Climbers to Squat Hops
FRIDAY—PULL	**A** Wide Grip Push-ups **B** Single Leg Static Lunges—left leg **C** High Knee High Arm Sprints in Place	**A** Bent Over Mid-Row (palms in) + Squat Hold **B** Single Leg Static Lunges—right leg **C** 10 Count Up Down	**A** Single Leg Dead Lift **B** 3 in 1 Lunge **C** Burpees with Weight	**A** Hammer Curls— heavy (both) **C** High Knee High Arm Sprints in Place **B** Side Plank Dips—left	**A** Biceps Curls—heavy (both) **C** 10 Count Up Downs **B** Side Plank Dips— right	**C** Burpees with Weight **C** High Knee High Arm Sprints in Place **C** 10 Count Up Downs
SATURDAY	1-Hour Cardio H.I.I.T. or SS (LSD)					
SUNDAY	Active Rest Day					

Pete Thomas's Lose It Fast 12-Week Workout Plan

LOSE IT FAST WORKOUT—WEEK 10

	Circuit 1	Circuit 2	Circuit 3	Circuit 4	Circuit 5	Cardio Circuit
MONDAY—PUSH	**A** Push-ups Rotate to Side Arm Raise **B** Squat Hops (4 Square) **C** Paper Plate Pushes	**A** Heavy DB Chest Flys **B** Squat to Rear Leg Lifts **C** 10 Count Mountain Climber to Squat Hops	**A** Punches with Dumbbells **B** Squat Hold with Skateboarders Kick **C** Burpees	**A** Overhead DB Triceps Presses—heavy **C** Paper Plate Pushes **B** Plank to Pointer (opposite arm opposite leg reach)	**A** Alternating Triceps Kick Backs—heavy **C** 10 Count Mountain Climbers to Squat Hops **B** Frog Sit-ups	**C** Burpees **C** Paper Plate Pushes **C** 10 Count Mountain Climbers to Squat Hops
TUESDAY—PULL	**A** Wide Grip Push-ups **B** Single Leg Static Lunge—left leg **C** High Knee High Arm Sprints in Place	**A** Bent Over Mid-Row (palms in) + Squat Hold **B** Single Leg Static Lunges—right leg **C** 10 Count Up Down	**A** Single Leg Dead Lifts **B** 3 in 1 Lunges **C** Burpees with Weight	**A** Hammer Curls Heavy (both) **C** High Knee High Arm Sprints in Place **B** Side Plank Dips—left	**A** Biceps Curls Heavy (both) **C** 10 Count Up Downs **B** Side Plank Dips—right	**C** Burpees with Weight **C** High Knee High Arm Sprints in Place **C** 10 Count Up Downs
WEDNESDAY	1- Hour Cardio H.I.I.T. or SS (LSD)					
THURSDAY—PUSH	**A** Push-ups Rotate to Side Arm Raises **B** Squat Hops (4 Square) **C** Paper Plate Pushes	**A** Heavy DB Chest Flys **B** Squat to Rear Leg Lifts **C** 10 Count Mountain Climber to Squat Hops	**A** Punches with Dumbbells **B** Squat Holds with Skateboarders Kick **C** Burpees	**A** Overhead DB Triceps Presses (heavy) **C** Paper Plate Pushes **B** Plank to Pointer (opposite arm opposite leg reach)	**A** Alternating Triceps Kick Backs—Heavy **C** 10 Count Mountain Climbers to Squat Hops **B** Frog Sit-ups	**C** Burpees **C** Paper Plate Pushes **C** 10 Count Mountain Climbers to Squat Hops
FRIDAY—PULL	**A** Wide Grip Push-ups **B** Single Leg Static Lunges—left leg **C** High Knee High Arm Sprints in Place	**A** Bent Over Mid-Row (palms in) + Squat Hold **B** Single Leg Static Lunges—right leg **C** 10 Count Up Downs	**A** Single Leg Dead Lifts **B** 3 in 1 Lunges **C** Burpees with Weight	**A** Hammer Curls Heavy (both) **C** High Knee High Arm Sprints in Place **B** Side Plank Dips—left	**A** Biceps Curls Heavy (both) **C** 10 Count Up Downs **B** Side Plank Dips—right	**C** Burpees with Weight **C** High Knee High Arm Sprints in Place **C** 10 Count Up Downs
SATURDAY	One Hour Cardio H.I.I.T. or SS (LSD)					
SUNDAY	Active Rest Day					

Pete Thomas's Lose It Fast 12-Week Workout Plan

LOSE IT FAST WORKOUT—WEEK 11

	Circuit 1	Circuit 2	Circuit 3	Circuit 4	Circuit 5	Cardio Circuit
MONDAY—PUSH	**A** Knee to Elbow Push-ups **B** Sumo Squat Jacks **C** 5 Step Floor Touches (Suicides)	**A** Plank to Push-ups **B** Weighted Goblet Squats **C** Burpees	**A** Squat to Shoulder Press (Thrusters) **B** Squat to Rear Leg Lunges **C** 10 Count Butt Kicks (both)	**A** Military (Triceps) Push-ups **C** 5 Step Floor Touches (Suicides) **B** Plank Hold + Punch	**A** Triceps Push-up Hold **C** Burpees **B** Reverse Hip Raises	**C** 10 Count Butt Kicks (double) **C** 5 Step Floor Touches (Suicides) **C** Burpees
TUESDAY—PULL	**A** Plank to DB Rows—left **B** Static Lunges—left leg **C** 10 Count Mountain Climbers + Squat Hops	**A** Plank to DB Row—right **B** Static Lunge—right leg **C** Burpees with Weight	**A** Plank to Squat **B** Jumping Switch Lunge **C** 10 Count Knee Tuck Jumps	**A** Biceps Curls with Squat Hold **C** 10 Count Mountain Climbers + Squat Hops **B** Weighted Ab Twists	**A** Biceps Curls to Shoulder Press **C** Burpees with Weight **B** Hip Raises with a Twist	**C** 10 Count Knee Tuck Jumps **C** 10 Count Mountain Climbers + Squat Hops **C** Burpees with Weight
WEDNESDAY	1-Hour Cardio H.I.I.T. or SS (LSD)					
THURSDAY—PUSH	**A** Knee to Elbow Push-ups **B** Sumo Squat Jacks **C** 5 Step Floor Touches (Suicides)	**A** Plank to Push-ups **B** Weighted Goblet Squats **C** Burpees	**A** Squat to Shoulder Press (Thrusters) **B** Squat to Rear Leg Lunges **C** 10 Count Butt Kicks (both)	**A** Military (Triceps) Push-ups **C** 5 Step Floor Touches (Suicides) **B** Plank Hold + Punch	**A** Triceps Push-ups Hold **C** Burpees **B** Reverse Hip Raises	**C** 10 Count Butt Kicks (Double) **C** 5 Step Floor Touches (Suicides) **C** Burpees
FRIDAY—PULL	**A** Plank to DB Row—left **B** Static Lunge—left leg **C** 10 Count Mountain Climbers + Squat Hops	**A** Plank to DB Row—right **B** Static Lunge—right leg **C** Burpees with Weight	**A** Plank to Squat **B** Jumping Switch Lunges **C** 10 Count Knee Tuck Jumps	**A** Biceps Curls with Squat Hold **C** 10 Count Mountain Climbers + Squat Hops **B** Weighted Ab Twists	**A** Biceps Curls to Shoulder Press **C** Burpees with Weight **B** Hip Raise with a Twist	**C** 10 Count Knee Tuck Jumps **C** 10 Count Mountain Climbers + Squat Hops **C** Burpees with Weight
SATURDAY	1-Hour Cardio H.I.I.T. or SS (LSD)					
SUNDAY	Active Rest Day					

Pete Thomas's Lose It Fast 12-Week Workout Plan

LOSE IT FAST WORKOUT—WEEK 12

	Circuit 1	Circuit 2	Circuit 3	Circuit 4	Circuit 5	Cardio Circuit
MONDAY—PUSH	**A** Knee to Elbow Push-ups **B** Sumo Squat Jacks **C** 5 Step Floor Touches (Suicides)	**A** Plank to Push-ups **B** Weighted Goblet Squats **C** Burpees	**A** Squat to Shoulder Press (Thrusters) **B** Squat to Rear Leg Lunges **C** 10 Count Butt Kicks (both)	**A** Military (Triceps) Push-ups **C** 5 Step Floor Touches (Suicides) **B** Plank Hold + Punch	**A** Triceps Push-ups Hold **C** Burpees **B** Reverse Hip Raises	**C** 10 Count Butt Kicks (double) **C** 5 Step Floor Touches (Suicides) **C** Burpees
TUESDAY—PULL	**A** Plank to DB Row—left **B** Static Lunges—left leg **C** 10 Count Mountain Climbers + Squat Hops	**A** Plank to DB Row—right **B** Static Lunge—right leg **C** Burpees with Weight	**A** Plank to Squat **B** Jumping Switch Lunge **C** 10 Count Knee Tuck Jumps	**A** Biceps Curls with Squat Hold **C** 10 Count Mountain Climbers + Squat Hops **B** Weighted Ab Twists	**A** Biceps Curls to Shoulder Press **C** Burpees with Weight **B** Hip Raises with a Twist	**C** 10 Count Knee Tuck Jumps **C** 10 Count Mountain Climbers + Squat Hops **C** Burpees with Weight
WEDNESDAY	1-Hour Cardio H.I.I.T. or SS (LSD)					
THURSDAY—PUSH	**A** Knee to Elbow Push-ups **B** Sumo Squat Jacks **C** 5 Step Floor Touches (Suicides)	**A** Plank to Push-ups **B** Weighted Goblet Squats **C** Burpees	**A** Squat to Shoulder Press (Thrusters) **B** Squat to Rear Leg Lunges **C** 10 Count Butt Kicks (both)	**A** Military (Triceps) Push-ups **C** 5 Step Floor Touches (Suicides) **B** Plank Hold + Punch	**A** Triceps Push-ups Hold **C** Burpees **B** Reverse Hip Raises	**C** 10 Count Butt Kicks (double) **C** 5 Step Floor Touches (Suicides) **C** Burpees
FRIDAY—PULL	**A** Plank to DB Row—left **B** Static Lunge—left leg **C** 10 Count Mountain Climbers + Squat Hops	**A** Plank to DB Row—right **B** Static Lunge—right leg **C** Burpees with Weight	**A** Plank to Squat **B** Jumping Switch Lunge **C** 10 Count Knee Tuck Jumps	**A** Biceps Curls with Squat Hold **C** 10 Count Mountain Climbers + Squat Hops **B** Weighted Ab Twists	**A** Biceps Curl to Shoulder Press **C** Burpees with Weight **B** Hip Raises with a Twist	**C** 10 Count Knee Tuck Jumps **C** 10 Count Mountain Climbers + Squat Hops **C** Burpees with Weight

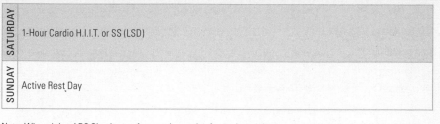

SATURDAY	1-Hour Cardio H.I.I.T. or SS (LSD)
SUNDAY	Active Rest Day

Note: When doing ABC Circuits, perform each exercise for 1 minute, then move to the next exercise in order. After you complete all three exercises in order (one circuit), then start over until you complete the circuit three times. Then move to the next circuit.

DESCRIPTIONS OF EXERCISES

A—Above the Waist

BICEPS

Biceps Curls Right / Left Arm

1. Stand with your feet shoulder-width apart. Grasp the dumbbells with palms facing forward and allow your arms to hang down at the sides. Elbows should be close to sides.
2. Flex the elbows and curl the dumbbells up to approximately shoulder level. Keep the elbows close to your sides throughout the movement.
3. Return to the start position.

Biceps Curls—21s 7 Low, 7 Hi, 7 Full

1. Stand with your feet shoulder-width apart, knees slightly bent.
2. Grasp the dumbbells in regular biceps curl manner and start with your arms hanging down.
3. For the first seven reps, bring the dumbbells up only to the midway point and return to the starting point.
4. For the next seven reps, start the movement at the midway point of the curl but bring the weight all the way to the shoulder, returning to the midway point to begin the next rep.
5. For the final seven reps, start the curl at the regular hanging position and bring the weight all the way to the shoulder for seven full reps.

Biceps Curls—Double

This is a regular biceps curl but done with both arms at the same time.

Biceps Curl—Double—Heavy Weight

These biceps curls use heavier weights with fewer reps, with both arms at the same time.

Biceps Curl to Shoulder Press

1. Stand with your feet shoulder-width apart.
2. Raise the dumbbells, curling them to your shoulders.
3. Turn your arms out (palms facing forward) to the shoulder press position. Lift the weights until your arms are fully extended, then return them to the original position by your side, and repeat.

Biceps Curl with Squat Hold

1. Start by holding a dumbbell in each hand.
2. Get into a squat position and hold for the whole exercise. Curl the dumbbells to shoulder level, then back down.
3. Return to the start position (hold the squat until done) and repeat.

Concentration Curls Right / Left Arm on One Knee

1. Sitting down on a bench or chair with your legs slightly apart, rest your elbow on the inside of your leg, just above your knee.
2. Hold the dumbbell palm forward and let your arm hang down in between your legs.
3. Curl the dumbbell up to shoulder level, then return to the start position.

Hammer Curls

1. Stand with feet shoulder-width apart and knees slightly bent.
2. Grasp the dumbbells with palms facing each other and allow your arms to hang down at the sides. Elbows should be close to your sides.
3. Flex at the elbows and curl the dumbbells up to approximately shoulder level. Keep your elbows close to your sides throughout the movement.

Hammer Curls—Alternating Fast Speed

1. These are hammer curls done with both arms.
2. Bring the dumbbells to the shoulder at a rapid speed, alternating arms.

Hammer Curls—Heavy

These hammer curls use heavier weights with fewer reps.

Reverse Grip Curls

1. Start with less weight than you would use for a regular biceps curl. Take a shoulder-width grip on the dumbbells, palms facing down (reversed from a normal curl).
2. Keeping your elbows close to your sides, knees slightly bent, curl it up as you would with a regular biceps curl. Hold for a second or two and then lower the weight slowly.

CHEST

DB Chest Press on Floor

1. Lie on the floor, facing the ceiling.
2. Hold a dumbbell in each hand with your arms extended up.
3. Bend your elbows and lower the dumbbells down toward your chest. Keep your elbows at 90 degrees and your wrists directly above your elbows.
4. Push up to return to the start position.

Dumbbell Chest Flys

1. Lie on your back on a bench or the ground. Bring the dumbbells to your shoulders. Press the dumbbells up directly above the chest with the dumbbells almost touching and palms facing each other.
2. Keeping the elbows slightly bent, lower the dumbbells out and away from each other in an arcing motion with hands aligned with the chest.
3. Let the upper arm go parallel to the ground before returning to the start position.

Dumbbell Pec Deck

1. Stand with your feet shoulder-width apart. Grasp the dumbbells and hold them directly overhead, with palms facing each other and elbows at 90 degrees.
2. Move your elbows toward each other in front of your body while maintaining the 90-degree angle. Try to bring the dumbbells as close to each other as possible. Return to the start position.

Explosive Push-up from Knees

1. Start by getting into a push-up position on your knees.
2. Lower your body to the ground and then explosively push up so that your hands leave the ground.
3. Catch your fall with your hands and immediately lower your body into a push-up again. Repeat.

Heavy Dumbbell Chest Flys

1. Lie on your back on a bench or the ground. Bring the heavy dumbbells to your shoulders. Press the dumbbells up directly above your chest with the dumbbells almost touching and palms facing each other.
2. Keeping the elbows slightly bent, lower the dumbbells out and away from each other in an arcing motion with hands aligned with the chest.
3. Let the upper arm go parallel to the ground before returning to the start position.

Heavy DB Chest Press

1. Lie on your back on the floor.
2. Hold a heavy dumbbell in each hand with arms extended up.
3. Bend your elbows and lower the dumbbells down toward your chest. Keep your elbows at 90 degrees and wrists directly above elbows.
4. Push up to return to the start position.

Knee to Elbow Push-ups

1. Lie facedown on the floor with your hands palms down, fingers pointing straight ahead, hands aligned with your chest.
2. Place your hands slightly wider than shoulder-width, and feet at hip-width with toes on the floor.
3. Extend the elbows and raise the body off the floor, bring your left knee up to your left elbow, then return.
4. Lower your entire body 4 to 8 inches from the floor.
5. Return to the start position by extending at the elbows and pushing the body up, bring your right knee to your right elbow, then return.

6. Keep the head and trunk stabilized in a neutral position by contracting the abdominal and back muscles. Never fully lock out the elbows at the start position and avoid hyperextension of the lower back.

Modified Push-up from Knees—Fast

1. Start by lying facedown and placing your hands near your shoulders with elbows pointing up.
2. Keeping your trunk straight, press your hands into the floor so that your upper body and hips come up off the ground into a push-up position. Knees remain on the floor.
3. Bend your elbows so that your chest touches the ground, and then repeat by returning to the top position. Do this as fast as possible.

Plank to Push-up

1. Get on the floor in modified plank with your forearms on the ground and your elbows aligned under your shoulders. Balance on your toes or knees.
2. Straighten your left arm, then the right. Hold full plank pose for 2 counts, then lower your left forearm, followed by the right, to the floor.
3. Repeat, switching the starting arm.

Push-up

1. Lie facedown on the floor with your hands palms down, fingers pointing straight ahead, hands aligned with your chest.
2. Place your hands slightly wider than shoulder-width, and feet at hip-width with your toes on the floor.
3. Extend your elbows and raise your body off the floor.
4. Lower your entire body 4 to 8 inches from the floor.
5. Return to the start position by extending at the elbows and pushing your body up.
6. Keep your head and trunk stabilized in a neutral position by contracting the abdominal and back muscles. Never fully lock out the elbows at the start position and avoid hyperextension of the lower back.

Push-up to Side Arm Raise

1. Lie facedown on the floor with hands palms down, fingers pointing straight ahead. Hands are aligned with your chest.
2. Place your hands slightly wider than shoulder-width, and feet at hip-width with your toes on floor.
3. Extend your elbows and raise your body off the floor, raising your left arm out to the side.
4. Replace your hand and lower your entire body 4 to 8 inches from the floor.
5. Return to the start position by extending at the elbows and pushing your body up, raising your right arm out to the side.
6. Keep your head and trunk stabilized in a neutral position by contracting the abdominal and back muscles. Never fully lock out the elbows at the start position and avoid hyperextension of the lower back.

Triangle Push-ups

1. Assume a push-up position, but form a triangular space with your hands under your chest by placing the tips of your index fingers together while doing the same with your thumbs.
2. Lower your chest to your hands, pause, and push back up.

LOWER BACK
Dumbbell—Kettle Bell—Swing

1. Stand straight with your legs shoulder-width apart.
2. Lean forward at your waist and go into a semi-squat. Your head faces forward and your back is straight.
3. Let your arms hang loose and raise the weight with both hands over your head.
4. Swing the weight with both hands between your legs (toward your back).
5. Thrust your hips forward to bring your weight back to the start position (it should be a fluid motion).
6. Repeat for specified time.

Heavy Dumbbell Dead Lift

1. Bend forward at the waist, pointing your arms straight down toward the floor. Maintain a slight natural curve in your lower back, and don't lock your knees.
2. Hold your dumbbells at arm's length, with your palms facing in.
3. Straighten your back slowly to a standing position, making sure not to lock your knees. Keep the dumbbells hanging gently at arm's length.
4. Lower yourself back to the start position.

Plank to Squat

1. Begin in plank (push-up) position, hands under shoulders.
2. Lower your body close to the ground. Keep your elbows close to your body, maintaining plank position.
3. Explode through the arms. Swing your feet under your chest to land evenly on both feet in a squatting position.

Single Legged Dead Lift

1. Bend forward at the waist, balancing on one leg, and pointing your arms straight down toward the floor. Maintain a slight natural curve in the lower back, and don't lock your knee.
2. Hold your dumbbells at arm's length, with your palms facing in.
3. Straighten your back slowly to a standing position, making sure not to lock your knee. Keep the dumbbells hanging gently at arm's length.
4. Lower yourself back to your start position. Repeat on the other leg.

Supermans

1. Lie on your stomach.
2. Simultaneously raise your legs up with your arms.
3. Return to the start position.

Weighted Supermans

1. Lie on your stomach.
2. Grab a dumbbell with both hands.
3. Simultaneously raise your legs up with your arms with the dumbbell.
4. Return to the start position.

SHOULDERS
Anterior Raise

1. Stand with your feet shoulder-width apart.
2. Grasp the dumbbells with palms down. Your arms should hang down in front of your body with your elbows slightly bent.
3. Raise the dumbbells to the front of your body at shoulder height, keeping your elbows only slightly bent.
4. Return to the start position.

Dumbbell Punches

1. Stand with your feet hip-width apart. Hold dumbbells in each hand.
2. Lift your arms to fighting stance and punch your arms out one at a time.
3. Repeat.

Dumbbell Shoulder Press

1. Stand with your feet shoulder-width apart and the dumbbells at shoulder level.
2. Press the dumbbells up above your head.
3. Return to the start position and repeat.

Lateral Raise

1. Stand with your feet hip-width apart. Hold dumbbells in each hand.
2. Lift your arms straight out to the sides in a lateral lift.
3. Return to the start position.

Squat to Shoulder Press Thrusters (alternate arms if necessary)

1. Start by holding the dumbbells at shoulder level.
2. Proceed into a full squat, and as you start to stand up, push the dumbbells overhead until fully extended.
3. Bring the dumbbells back down to shoulder level and repeat.

Vertical Row (Zippers)

1. Stand with your feet hip-width apart. Hold dumbbells in each hand.
2. Lift your arms straight up your body (as if you are pulling up a zipper).
3. Return to the start position.

TRICEPS
Overhead Triceps Press • Right / Left • Double Arm

1. Stand with your feet shoulder-width apart. Grasp the dumbbells and press them directly overhead, palms facing each other.
2. Stabilize your shoulders and lower the weight, moving only at the elbow joint until your forearms are parallel to the floor. Keep your elbows pointing forward throughout the movement.
3. Return to the start position.

Push-up Hold

1. Get into the push-up position on the floor with your hands under your shoulders and your body in a straight line (plank) position.
2. Drop down, maintaining a straight line in your body. When you get to the bottom of the position just above the floor, hold the position for a few seconds.
3. Push yourself back up to the start position and repeat. Maintain a straight line by keeping a tight core throughout the exercise.

Triceps Kick Backs • Right / Left • Double Arm

1. This exercise can be done kneeling on a bench with an arm supporting your weight, or on your feet bent over until your torso is parallel to the floor. Keep the abs engaged to support the lower back.
2. Holding a dumbbell in one or both hands, bring your elbows up to torso level so that your upper arm is parallel to the floor and your arm is at a 90-degree angle.
3. Straighten the arm(s) out behind you, squeezing the triceps muscles. The arm(s) should be straight with your palm facing inward toward your body.
4. Bend the arms back to the start position and repeat. Keep the abs engaged and the back flat throughout the movement.

Triceps (Military) Push-ups

1. Get into a plank/push-up position, with your elbows close to your body.
2. Lower your body to the ground; elbows should move straight back, not flare outward. Be sure to maintain the plank position.

3. If this movement is too difficult, do a regression of the push-ups using your knees at first.

Triceps Skull Crushers

1. Lie on a flat bench face-up with legs on each side on the floor.
2. Hold a single dumbbell with both hands above your chest (or use two if they are lighter), straight up, with the dumbbell shaft parallel to the floor.
3. Move the weight down toward the rear of your head with a flexing of the elbows. Continue lowering the weight behind the head until the dumbbell head is about in line with the bench top, or a little higher if that feels unstable. Some people, if they are using two dumbbells, bring the weights down to the side of their ears instead of to the rear of the head.
4. Reverse the movement until the weight is held above the chest and repeat.

UPPER BACK

Bent Over Flys

1. Hold a dumbbell in each hand with palms facing each other and arms straight.
2. Bend forward at the waist, keeping your back straight, until your back is parallel to the floor.
3. Keeping your elbows slightly bent, squeeze your shoulder blades together and raise your forearms and the dumbbells out to the side toward the ceiling as if you were flapping imaginary wings, stopping at shoulder level. Lower down slowly.

Bent Over Mid-Row—Palms In (with Squat Hold)

1. With a dumbbell in each hand (palms facing your torso), bend your knees slightly and bring your torso forward by bending at the waist; as you bend make sure to keep your back straight until it is almost parallel to the floor.
2. While keeping the torso stationary, squat down and lift the dumbbells to your sides, keeping the elbows close to the body. At the top position, squeeze the back muscles and hold for a second.

3. Slowly lower the weight to the start position, staying in squat position during whole exercise.

Bent Over Y Raise

1. Grab a pair of dumbbells, bend at your hips, and lower your torso until it's nearly parallel to the floor. Let your arms hang straight from your shoulders, and slightly bend your knees.
2. Now raise your arms so they're at a 30-degree angle to your body (forming a Y) and are in line with your torso. Pause, lower, and repeat.

Dumbbell High Row (overhead)

1. Hold a dumbbell in each hand with palms facing back and arms straight.
2. Bend forward at the waist, keeping your back straight, until your back is parallel to the floor.
3. With your elbows bent and facing the ceiling, raise your elbows up while bringing the dumbbells toward your shoulders. Lower down slowly.

Dumbbell Low Row (underhand)

1. Hold dumbbells in each hand with palms facing each other. Bend forward at about a 45-degree angle and let your arms hang down.
2. With your elbows slightly bent and facing the ceiling, raise the dumbbells to your waist and squeeze your shoulder blades together at the top of the movement.
3. Return to the start position.

One Arm Overhead Dumbbell Snatch • Right / Left

1. Grab a light dumbbell in one hand and stand with your feet shoulder-width apart. Keeping your back flat, bend at the hips and knees as if you were in the start position of a dead lift, and let the hand with the dumbbell hang just below your knees.
2. Explosively jump up, extending your entire body so that you come up on your toes. As you rise, pull the weight straight up in front of your body until it reaches the middle of your chest, then invert the wrists and push the weight overhead—but don't let go.

3. Let the momentum generated in your hips move the dumbbell most of the way upward—don't just stand up and do a shoulder press.

One Arm Row

1. Bend over at your lower back, keeping your back flat.
2. Take one hand and grab a dumbbell. Rest the other hand on the opposite knee or a bench.
3. Row up toward your waist just like a bent over row.
4. Squeeze your shoulder blade in toward your spine when performing the row.

Plank to Row • Right / Left

1. Start by getting into a plank position and grip a dumbbell in one hand.
2. Holding this plank position, row the dumbbell up to chest level squeezing through your shoulder blades, and return to the floor.

Wide Grip Push-ups

1. Place your hands flat on the floor, wider than shoulder-width apart.
2. Lower your body down to the floor until your chest brushes the ground. Keep your elbows tucked in by your sides. Your elbows should go down and back, not flare out to the side.
3. Return to the start position.

B—Below or at the Waist

ABS—OBLIQUES

Bicycles (Speed)

1. Lie on your back with your knees bent at a 90-degree angle to the floor.
2. Place your hands behind your ears but do not pull on your neck.
3. Bring one knee to the opposite elbow, while pushing out with the opposite foot as if you were riding a bike.
4. Alternate sides.

Hip Raise with a Twist

1. Lie on your back with your legs lifted up toward the ceiling in line with your hips. Cross your legs at the ankles.

2. Extend your arms out from your body to the sides with fingertips pressed into the floor.
3. Slowly lift up with the hips, as if your legs are flat up against a wall and they can only move straight up. Avoid rolling forward or back.
4. Once your legs are straight above your waist, twist your hips once each direction.
5. Slowly return your hips to the floor and repeat.

Side Bends

1. Start in standing position, knees soft.
2. Hold dumbbells in your hands at your sides, and slowly bend to the side, lowering the weight toward the floor. Return to starting position.
3. Alternate sides.

Side Crunches with Knee over Knee
(elbow touches ground at bottom of crunch)

1. Lie with your back flat on the exercise mat. Bring your knees up into normal crunch position with your feet flat on the floor.
2. Cross one leg over the other. Your legs should form a sort of triangle.
3. Bring your hands behind your head so your fingertips just touch each other as they rest behind your head.
4. Bring your body up into a side crunch and touch your elbow to the opposite bent knee. Your side will bend as your shoulder lifts off the ground into the crunch.
5. Lower yourself gently back down on the mat. Repeat, switching sides regularly.

Side Heel Touches

1. Lie on your back with your knees bent and feet on the ground.
2. Place your hands palms down on the floor and slowly slide one hand down to one heel (keep your hand flat on the ground).
3. Alternate sides.

Side Plank Dip • Right / Left

1. Lie on your left side with your right foot crossed over the left and your right hand behind your head. Rest your left forearm on the floor

perpendicular to your body, elbow under shoulder. Lift your hips so your legs are off the floor, keeping your forearm on the floor for support.

2. Slowly lower your hips to 1 to 2 inches off the floor and return to the starting position. Repeat.

3. Switch sides and repeat.

Side Plank Hold • Right / Left

1. Lie on your left side with your right foot crossed over the left and right hand behind your head. Rest your left forearm on the floor perpendicular to your body, elbow under shoulder. Lift your hips so your legs are off the floor, keeping your forearm on the floor for support.

2. Raise your body using one forearm and side of feet. Support your body in this raised position and hold the position.

3. Switch sides and repeat.

Side Rows (legs off ground)

1. Sit on the ground with only your butt touching the floor, legs off the ground.

2. Row a dumbbell from side to side (like you are rowing a boat).

Weighted Cross Body Punch-ups

1. Lie on your back with your knees bent and feet on the ground.

2. Hold dumbbells in your hands and sit up.

3. Punch alternating sides while twisting at the waist, when all the way up.

4. Slowly lower back to the ground and repeat, starting the punch with the opposite arm.

Weighted Twists (Russian Twists)

1. Grab a dumbbell or weight plate and sit on the floor with your hips and knees bent 90 degrees.

2. Hold the weight straight out in front of you and keep your back straight (your torso should be at about 45 degrees to the floor). Explosively twist your torso as far as you can to the left and then reverse the motion, twisting as far as you can to the right.

ABS—RECTUS
Crunches

1. Lie on your back with your knees bent, feet flat on the floor.
2. Put your hands behind your head so that your thumbs are behind your ears.
3. Tilt your chin slightly, leaving a few inches of space between chin and chest.
4. Gently pull your abdominals inward.
5. Curl up and forward so that your head, neck, and shoulder blades are off the floor. Hold for a few seconds and then lower slowly back down. Do not pull on your neck.

Elbow to Raised Knee Crunch

1. Start by lying on your back with your hands behind your head.
2. Simultaneously curl your right shoulder and left knee up toward the center of your body until elbow and knee touch. Return to the start position and repeat with the other side.

Flutter Kicks

1. Lie on your back on the floor with your legs extended out in front of you and your abdominal muscles contracted.
2. Lift your head and shoulders slightly off the mat.
3. Lift your feet about six inches off the ground, and alternate kicking your left and right leg up and down in a rapid motion. Drop your feet closer to the ground to intensify the exercise, or kick higher if your back is arching or it's too challenging for you at this point.

Frog Sit-ups

1. Lie flat on the floor with your legs extended.
2. Bend your knees and turn your feet in so that the soles of your feet are touching. Pull the feet toward the thighs as much as possible.
3. Cross your arms in front of your chest so that your hands are touching the opposite shoulders.
4. Sit up while trying to touch your elbows to your knees or toes.
5. Return slowly to the original position and repeat.

Planks

1. Lie facedown on the floor with your hands palms down, fingers pointing straight ahead.
2. Drop your elbows to the floor directly under your shoulders. Raise the body off the floor onto your forearms and toes. Hold the position.

Plank to Punch

1. Start in plank position with your hands under your shoulders and legs extended outward.
2. Punch your right fist forward with force, returning the hand to the plank position. Alternate hands and repeat.

Plank with Opposite Leg Opposite Arm Reach (Pointers)

1. Start in a tabletop position (on both hands and knees), then raise your right arm to shoulder height as if pointing, at the same time straightening the left leg to hip height as if pointing backward with the toes.
2. Repeat with the opposite arm and leg.

Reverse Hip Raise

1. Lie on your back with your legs lifted up toward the ceiling in line with your hips. Cross your legs at the ankles.
2. Extend your arms out from your body to the sides with fingertips pressed into the floor.
3. Slowly lift up with the hips, as if your legs are flat up against a wall and they can only move straight up. Avoid rolling forward or back. Slowly return your hips to the floor and repeat.

Scissors

1. Lie down on the floor with your hands under your butt to reduce the strain on your lower back. Raise both legs 15 to 20 inches off the ground. Kick your legs outward like the opening of a scissors.
2. Bring your legs back to the center and cross them over each other (like closing a scissors).
3. Do the kick in alternating fashion, being sure to keep your abs flexed the entire time.

Sit-ups

1. Lie on the floor with your knees bent, hands behind your head (not clasped).
2. Tighten your abdominal muscles as you sit all the way up.
3. Return your body slowly to the start position and repeat.

V Sit-up—Knee to Chest / Rockers

1. Lie on the floor with your hands flat on the floor next to you.
2. Bring your knees and chest toward the center of your body (use your hands for support).
3. Extend your knees back out but do not let them touch the floor.
4. Rock your body back to the start position and repeat.

Weighted Sit-ups with Dumbbell on Chest

1. Lie on the floor with your knees bent, with a dumbbell held to your chest.
2. Tighten your abdominal muscles as you sit all the way up.
3. Return your body slowly to the original position and repeat.

LUNGES—HAMSTRING
3 in 1 Lunge

1. Stand with feet hip-width apart.
2. Step forward, lunging 2 to 3 feet and forming a 90-degree bend at the front hip and knee. Do not allow the front knee to extend past the toes. Return to the start position, without touching your foot to the ground.
3. Step the same foot backward 2 to 3 feet and lower your body, forming a 90-degree bend at the front hip and knee. Do not allow the front knee to extend past the toes.
4. Pushing off the front foot, return to the start position, without touching your foot to the ground.
5. Step the same foot out to the side 2 to 3 feet and lower the body to the side, forming a 90-degree bend at front hip and knee. Do not allow front knee to extend past the toes.
6. Return to the start position and repeat the same movements on the other side.

Forward Lunge with Kick

1. Stand with feet hip-width apart.
2. Step forward, lunging 2 to 3 feet, forming a 90-degree bend at the front hip and knee. Do not allow the front knee to extend past the toes.
3. Bring your back leg forward and kick it in front while balancing on the opposite leg.
4. Return your kicking leg to the start position.
5. Repeat with the opposite leg.

Jumping Switch (Plyo) Lunge

1. Stand in a split stance, right leg in front and left leg in back.
2. Bend your knees and lower into a lunge, keeping the front knee be-hind the toe. In an explosive movement, jump into the air and switch your legs, landing so that the left leg is in front and the right leg is in back.
3. Land with soft knees, lower into a lunge, and repeat, jumping and switching sides.

Lunge Hold Pulse

1. Start in a lunge position.
2. Hold the lunge for 30 seconds. Switch legs and hold for 30 seconds.

Lunge Hold Pulse to Rear Leg Lift

1. Start in a forward lunge position.
2. Hold the lunge for 30 seconds.
3. Return to the start position and lift your leg back.
4. Switch legs and repeat.

Lunge with Biceps Curl

1. Stand with feet hip-width apart. Hold dumbbells in each hand.
2. Step forward and lower your body, forming a 90-degree bend at the front hip and knee. Do not allow the front knee to extend past the toes. While lunging forward, lift your arms up into a biceps curl.
3. Return to the start position. Then lunge forward with other leg. Con-tinue alternating legs, doing biceps curls with each lunge.

Pelvic Thrust

1. Lie on the floor with your knees bent about hip-width apart, feet planted firmly on the floor. Place your hands palms down next to your hips.
2. Lift your body off of the ground while digging your heels into the floor. Only your shoulders and feet should be touching the ground.
3. Return to the start position.

Pelvic Thrust—One Leg

1. Lie on the floor with one foot on the floor about hip-width apart. Hold one leg out and place your hands palms down next to your hips.
2. Lift your body off the ground. Only your shoulders and one foot should be touching the ground.
3. Return to the start position and repeat on the other side.

Reverse Lunge

1. Stand with feet hip-width apart.
2. Step one foot backward 2 to 3 feet and lower your body, forming a 90-degree bend at the front hip and knee. Do not allow the front knee to extend past the toes.
3. Pushing off the front foot, return to the start position. Switch legs and repeat.

Reverse Lunge to Forward Knee Raise

1. Stand with feet hip-width apart.
2. Step one foot backward 2 to 3 feet and lower your body, forming a 90-degree bend at the front hip and knee. Do not allow the front knee to extend past the toes.
3. Pushing off the front foot, return to the start position and raise your back leg forward, raising your knee. Switch legs and repeat.

Reverse Lunge to Forward Knee Raise Hop

1. Stand with feet hip-width apart.
2. Step one foot backward 2 to 3 feet and lower your body, forming a 90-degree bend at the front hip and knee. Do not allow the front knee to extend past the toes.

3. Pushing off the front foot, return to the start position, raise your back leg forward, raise your knee and hop. Switch legs and repeat.

Side Lunge

1. Start by placing your feet in a wide stance.
2. Shift your weight and hips to one side and squat down so that your hips drop down behind that foot.
3. Return to the start position and repeat the same movement on the other side.

Single Leg Static Lunge / Right Leg

1. Stand with feet hip-width apart.
2. Step forward with your right leg, lunging 2 to 3 feet, forming a 90-degree bend at the front hip and knee. Do not allow the front knee to extend past the toes. Return to the start position.
3. Repeat with right leg.

Single Leg Static Lunge / Left Leg

1. Stand with feet hip-width apart.
2. Step forward with your left leg, lunging 2 to 3 feet, forming a 90-degree bend at the front hip and knee. Do not allow the front knee to extend past the toes. Return to the start position.
3. Repeat with left leg.

Static / Forward Lunge

1. Stand with feet hip-width apart.
2. Step forward, lunging 2 to 3 feet, forming a 90-degree bend at the front hip and knee. Do not allow the front knee to extend past the toes. Return to the start position. Repeat with the opposite leg.

Traveling Lunge

1. Stand with feet hip-width apart.
2. Step forward, lunging 2 to 3 feet, forming a 90-degree bend at the front hip and knee. Do not allow the front knee to extend past the toes.
3. Balancing on the front foot, bring the rear leg forward to the starting position, repeating the exercise on the opposite leg.

Weighted Forward Lunge

1. Stand with feet hip-width apart. Place dumbbells in your hands and hold on to them on the outside of your legs.
2. Step forward, lunging 2 to 3 feet, forming a 90-degree bend at the front hip and knee. Do not allow the front knee to extend past the toes. Lift back to the start position and bring the other leg forward, repeating the exercise on the opposite leg.

Weighted Forward Lunge with Side to Side Twist

1. Stand with feet hip-width apart. Grasp dumbbells and hold them out in front of your body.
2. Step forward 2 to 3 feet, forming a 90-degree bend at the front hip and knee. Do not allow the front knee to extend past the toes. As you are lunging, swing the dumbbells across your body toward the hip.
3. Pushing off the front foot, return to the start position with your legs and dumbbells. Continue with the same leg or alternate as prescribed.

SQUATS—QUADRICEPS

Air Squat

1. Stand with your feet slightly wider than hip-width apart. Knees should be slightly bent and arms out in front of the body.
2. Lower your body by flexing at the hips and knees. Sit back so that the knees do not go over the toes.
3. Once the thighs are parallel to the floor, return to the start position.

Deep Sumo Squat (sub 90 degrees)

1. Stand with your feet wider than shoulder-width and your toes pointed slightly outward.
2. Drop your hips back and down until you are in a sitting position and hips are below 90 degrees, while your knees stay directly above your feet.
3. Return to the start position and repeat.

Dumbbell Squat

1. Grasp dumbbells and let your arms hang down at the sides.
2. Stand with your feet slightly wider than hip-width apart. Knees should be slightly bent.
3. Lower your body by flexing at the hips and knees. Sit back and down so that the knees do not go over the toes.
4. Once your thighs are parallel to floor, return to the start position.

Goblet Squat

1. Start by holding a dumbbell with two hands against your chest at about shoulder level by placing the palms of your hands underneath one end of the dumbbell.
2. Your feet should be wider than shoulder-width and your toes pointed slightly outward.
3. Proceed to squat down while holding the dumbbells against your chest.
4. Your hips should drop back and down while your knees stay directly above your feet.
5. Return to the start position and repeat.

Jump Squat

1. Stand with your feet shoulder-width apart, trunk flexed forward slightly with back straight in a neutral position.
2. Your arms should be in the "ready" position, with elbows flexed at approximately 90 degrees.
3. Lower your body to where your thighs are parallel to the ground in a squatting position.
4. Jump up with your arms raising overhead.
5. Land on both feet. Repeat.

Prisoner Squat

1. Stand with your feet slightly wider than hip-width apart. Knees should be slightly bent and hands resting on the back of your head.
2. Lower your body by flexing at the hips and knees. Sit back so that the knees do not go over the toes.
3. Once your thighs are parallel to the floor, return to the start position.

Side to Side Squat

1. Start by placing your hands behind your head and your feet in a wide stance.
2. Shift your weight and hips to one side and squat down so that your hips drop down behind that foot.
3. Return to the start position and repeat the same movement on the other side.

Squat Holds

1. Stand with your feet wider than shoulder-width and your toes pointed slightly outward.
2. Drop your hips back and down while your knees stay directly above your feet.
3. Hold squat position.

Squat Hold with Skateboard Rear Kick

1. Stand with your feet wider than shoulder-width and your toes pointed slightly outward.
2. Drop your hips back and down while your knees stay directly above your feet.
3. Kick out behind you like you are riding a skateboard.

Squat Hop 4 Square

1. Stand with your feet slightly wider than hip-width apart. Knees should be slightly bent and hands are resting at the back of your head.
2. Lower your body by flexing at the hips and knees. Sit back so that the knees do not go over the toes.
3. Once your thighs are parallel to the floor, hop up and turn 90 degrees (while hopping). Repeat 4 times (in the shape of a square).

Squat to Rear Leg Lift

1. Stand with your feet hip-width apart, arms at your sides.
2. Cross your right leg behind your left, slightly left of your left heel, and rest your toe on the floor about 2 feet behind you.
3. Keeping your right heel up, squat down as far as you can without letting your left knee extend past your toes.

4. Straighten your left leg and raise your right leg as high as possible behind you, lowering your torso toward the floor.
5. Return to the start position.

Squat to Rear Leg Lunge

1. Stand with your feet shoulder-width apart, arms at your sides, and lower your butt until your thighs are parallel to the ground. Push back up to the start position. Next, take a giant step back with your left foot and lower your body until your right thigh is parallel to the ground.
2. Push up with your right leg while curling your left heel toward your glutes. That's 1 rep. Repeat.

Squat with a Front Kick

1. Stand with your feet together and fists up, protecting your face.
2. Bring your right knee up and extend the leg in a front kick, without fully extending the knee.
3. Lower the leg and bend your knees into a low squat (knees behind toes) and then stand and kick with the left leg. Repeat (right kick, squat, left kick).

Sumo Squat

1. Stand with your feet wider than shoulder-width and your toes pointed slightly outward.
2. Drop your hips back and down while your knees stay directly above your feet.
3. Return to the start position and repeat.

Weighted Squat with a Punch

1. Stand with your feet slightly wider than hip-width apart. Knees should be slightly bent.
2. Grasp dumbbells and hold them next to your chest.
3. Lower your body by flexing at the hips and knees. Sit back so that the knees do not go over the toes.
4. Once your thighs are parallel to the floor, punch out your arms (one at a time), then return to the start position.

C—Cardio

5 Step Floor Touch (Suicides)

1. Stand with your feet together and knees slightly bent. Quickly run to the right 5 steps and touch the floor.
2. Quickly run to the left 5 steps and touch the floor.
3. Repeat.

Burpees

1. From a standing position, jump as high as possible, land down on your feet, and place your hands on the ground in front of your feet.
2. Hop your feet back into a push-up position, perform a push-up, then hop forward and jump back up again as fast as possible.

Burpees with Dumbbell

1. From a standing position, jump as high as possible with weights in your hands, land down on your feet, and place your hands on your dumbbells on the ground in front of your feet.
2. Hop your feet back into a push-up position, then hop back forward and up again as fast as possible.

Butt Kicks

Jog in place while lifting your heels toward your butt with every step.

10 Count Double Butt Kicks

1. Jog in place while lifting your heels toward your butt with every step for a count of 10.
2. Lift both legs at the same time, kicking yourself in the butt with both knees.
3. Repeat.

Cross Arm Jacks

1. Start with your legs side by side and your arms by your sides.
2. Perform a jumping jack but cross one arm over the midpoint of your body while crossing your leg in a scissor motion.
3. Repeat with the other arm.

Cross-Country Skiers Switch Feet

1. Jump straight legs forward and back while swinging opposite arms front and back.
2. Alternate sides.

Fast Feet Hot Feet

Run in place, swinging your arms as fast as possible.

Heismans (1-2-3 Knee Up)

1. Stand with your feet together and knees slightly bent. Arms should be bent at the elbow.
2. Take three quick steps to the right while swinging your arms.
3. Balance on your right foot while lifting your left leg and knee up to your chest, squeezing your abs and extending your left arm so that it is pointing at your left foot.
4. Repeat in the opposite direction.

High Knees

1. Stand in place with your feet hip-width apart.
2. Lift your knee up toward your chest and quickly place the foot back on the ground. Repeat with the other knee. Keep a fast pace with minimal ground contact time.

High Knee Sprints (High Arm)

1. Stand in place with your feet hip-width apart.
2. Lift your knee up toward your chest and quickly place the foot back on the ground, swinging the opposite arm high at the same time. Repeat with the other knee and arm. Keep a fast pace with minimal ground contact time.

Ice Skaters with Hop

1. Start with your feet a little wider than shoulder-width apart. Bend your knees and lean forward slightly with your arms at your sides.
2. Shift your weight to your left leg. Jump 3 feet to the right, landing on your right foot. Your left foot should lift and come near your right ankle, but it should not touch the ground. Jump again, this time

landing on your left foot; bring your right foot near your left ankle, but do not touch the floor. Swing your arms to help with balance and increase the length of your jumps.

3. Repeat.

Jog in Place • Jump Rope

1. Start with a real or imaginary jump rope in each hand.
2. Jump off the ground and start swinging the real or imaginary jump rope under your feet.
3. Continue jumping up and down as you bring the jump rope under your feet.

Jumping Jacks

1. Start with your legs side by side and your arms by your sides.
2. In one motion, jump and spread your legs out to the sides while you raise your arms out and up over your head. Land in this position and then return to the start position.

10 Count Knee Tuck Jumps

1. Begin standing with your knees slightly bent.
2. Quickly squat a short distance, flexing the hips and knees, and immediately extend to jump for maximum vertical height.
3. As you go up, flex your hips and bring your knees forward and upward, attempting to touch the chest with the knees.
4. Finish the motion by landing with your knees only partially bent, using your legs to absorb the impact.
5. Perform quick feet for a count of 10. Repeat.

Mountain Climbers

1. Start by getting on your hands and feet in a prone position.
2. Keeping your body parallel to ground, alternate jumping your knees toward your chest.
3. Repeat.

10 Count Mountain Climber Squat Hops

1. Start by getting on your hands and feet in a prone position.
2. Keeping your body parallel to the ground, alternate bringing your knees toward your chest.
3. After 10 counts, hop both legs toward your chest, go into the squat position, and hop up.
4. Place your hands back on the ground and kick your legs back into the push-up position. Repeat.

Plank to Squat

1. Begin in plank (push-up) position, hands under shoulders.
2. Lower your body close to the ground. Keep your elbows close to your body, maintaining plank position.
3. Explode through the arms. Swing your feet under your chest to land evenly on both feet in a squatting position.

Side to Side Donkey Kicks

1. Get on your hands and knees on the floor.
2. Keeping your knee at a 90-degree angle, raise your right leg, keeping your weight on your left knee.
3. Keep your back straight and do not lean backward or forward. Do not raise your right thigh and knee above the line of your back or neck. Your right foot should be pointing toward the ceiling.
4. Lower your right leg back to the start position. Repeat with your left leg.

Side Jump (Side-to-Side Hops)

1. Imagine an invisible line on the ground.
2. Stand on one side of the invisible line, then jump to the other side of the line, landing on both feet. Jump back and forth over the line.

Squat Hops

1. Stand with your feet shoulder-width apart, trunk flexed forward slightly with your back straight in a neutral position.
2. Your arms should be in the "ready" position with elbows flexed at approximately 90 degrees.
3. Lower your body to where your thighs are parallel to the ground.

4. Jump up, raising your arms overhead.
5. Land on both feet.

10 Count Squat Hops

1. Stand with your feet shoulder-width apart, trunk flexed forward slightly with your back straight in a neutral position.
2. Your arms should be in the "ready" position with elbows flexed at approximately 90 degrees.
3. Lower your body to where the thighs are parallel to the ground.
4. Jump up, raising your arms overhead.
5. Land on both feet.
6. Do 10 counts of quick feet. Repeat.

Straight Arm Jumping Jacks

1. Start with your legs side by side and your hands clasped at your chest.
2. In one motion, jump and spread your legs out to the sides while your arms raise straight up above your head. Land in this position and then return to the start position.

Sumo Jacks

1. Position your legs in sumo stance, hands out. Stay low and keep your weight back with a good squat position
2. Hop your legs inward without raising your body.
3. Hop your legs outward without raising your body.

Towel / Paper Plate Pushes

1. Place a towel or paper plate on a smooth floor. Place your hands on the towel or paper plate.
2. While bending down, push the towel or plate across the floor, keeping your hands on the towel or paper plate at all times.

5 Count Up Downs

1. Do 5 counts of quick feet.
2. After 5 counts of quick feet, drop to the floor and perform a standard push-up.

3. After you complete the push-up, return to your standing position and repeat the sequence.

10 Count Up Downs

1. Do 10 counts of quick feet.
2. After 10 counts of quick feet, drop to the floor and perform a standard push-up.
3. After you complete the push-up, return to your standing position and repeat the sequence.

Wall Sit

1. Place your back against the wall.
2. Proceed into a squat position so that your thighs are parallel to the ground.
3. Hold this position for 1 minute.

Weighted Jumping Jacks

1. Start with your legs side by side and your arms by your sides with weights.
2. In one motion, jump and spread your legs out to the sides while you raise your arms with weights, out and up overhead. Land in this position and then return to the start position.

SECONDARY WORKOUTS FOR "TWO-A-DAYS"

I've mentioned that if you really want to see rapid results, you can consider adding a second workout every day (except Sunday, your "active" rest day). The following list will provide these secondary workouts. They are listed in chronological order from weeks 1 to 4 to weeks 9 to 12, as follows:

■ Monday, Tuesday, Thursday, Friday Secondary Workouts (these are cardio workouts for your ABC Circuit days)
■ Wednesday and Saturday Primary Workouts (Cardio)
■ Wednesday and Saturday Secondary Workouts (Cardio)

Believe me, if you include these secondary workouts into your routine, you will certainly Lose It Fast!

PURSUIT PHASE

Secondary Workouts for Monday/Tuesday/Thursday/Friday and Saturday, and Primary Workout for Wednesday/Saturday

WEEKS 1 TO 4

MONDAY/TUESDAY/THURSDAY/FRIDAY—SECONDARY WORKOUT

BEGINNING 1 INTERVALS (ANY MACHINE)

5 minutes	Warm-up (HR = 70%)
:30 seconds	Up interval (HR = 85% and above)
4:30 minutes	Down interval (HR = 75% to 85%)
Next 50 minutes	Repeat
5 minutes	Cooldown (HR = 65%)

Or

BEGINNING 2 INTERVALS (ANY MACHINE)

5 minutes	Warm-up (HR = 70%)
1 minute	Up interval (HR – 05% and above)
4 minutes	Down interval (HR = 75% to 85%)
Next 50 minutes	Repeat
5 minutes	Cooldown (HR = 65%)

Or

PETE'S A.M. TREADMILL WORKOUT

Warm-up	
5 minutes	R = 70% (Incline 1—approx. speed 5.0)
Workout	
25 minutes	HR = 80% to 85% (Incline 2—approx. speed 5.5)
25 minutes	HR = 85% to 95% (Incline 2—approx speed 6.5)
Cooldown	
5 minutes	HR = 70% to 80% (Incline 1—approx speed 5.0)

WEEKS 1 TO 4
WEDNESDAY AND SATURDAY PRIMARY WORKOUT

PETE'S ALL-WALKING TREADMILL WORKOUT (TARGET HEART RATE AVERAGE—85%)

Warm-up	Warm-up (HR = 70%)
2 minutes	Incline 2—approx. speed 3.5
2 minutes	Incline 4—approx. speed 3.5
Workout	
2 minutes	Incline 6—approx. speed 3.5
2 minutes	Incline 8—approx. speed 3.5
2 minutes	Incline 10—approx. speed 3.5
2 minutes	Incline 12—approx. speed 3.5
2 minutes	Incline 15—approx. speed 3.5
Repeat for 50 minutes	
Warm down	
2 minutes	Incline 6—approx. speed 3.5
2 minutes	Incline 4—approx. speed 3.5
2 minutes	Incline 2—approx. speed 3.5
2 minutes	Incline 0—approx. speed 3.5

WEEKS 1 TO 4
WEDNESDAY AND SATURDAY SECONDARY WORKOUT

**PETE'S KICK-BUTT ELLIPTICAL WORKOUT
(TARGET HEART RATE AVERAGE—85% AND ABOVE)**
(This is for a Precor Elliptical 576i with incline and resistance. Modify for your machinery.)

Incline	Resistance	RPM	Time	Direction
10	10	100	10 minutes	Forward
10	10	90	10 minutes	Reverse
10	18	100	10 minutes	Forward
10	18	90	10 minutes	Reverse
5	3	120	10 minutes	Reverse
5	3	120	10 minutes	Forward

WEEKS 5 TO 8
MONDAY/TUESDAY/THURSDAY/FRIDAY SECONDARY WORKOUT

INTERMEDIATE INTERVALS (ANY MACHINE)

5 minutes	Warm-up (HR = 70%)
1 minute	Up interval (HR = 85% and above)
2 minutes	Down interval (HR = 75% to 85%)
Next 50 minutes	Repeat
5 minutes	Cooldown (HR = 65%)

WEEKS 5 TO 8
WEDNESDAY AND SATURDAY PRIMARY WORKOUT

PETE'S REGULAR ELLIPTICAL WORKOUT (TARGET HEART RATE AVERAGE—85%)

Resistance	RPM	Time	Direction
12	10.0	10 minutes	Forward
12	10.0	10 minutes	Reverse
18	7.0	10 minutes	Forward
18	7.0	10 minutes	Reverse
3	15.0	10 minutes	Reverse
3	15.0	10 minutes	Forward

WEEKS 5 TO 8
WEDNESDAY AND SATURDAY SECONDARY WORKOUT

PETE'S REGULAR TREADMILL WORKOUT

Warm-up	
5 minutes	HR = 70% to 80% (Incline 1—approx. speed 5.0)
Workout	
25 minutes	HR = 80% to 85% (Incline 2—approx. speed 5.5)
25 minutes	HR = 85% to 95% (Incline 2—approx. speed 6.5)
Cooldown	
5 minutes	HR = 70% to 80% (Incline 1—approx. speed 5.0)

WEEKS 9 TO 12
MONDAY/TUESDAY/THURSDAY/FRIDAY SECONDARY WORKOUT

TREADMILL INTERVALS

5 minutes	Warm-up—HR = 70% (Incline 0.5%—approx. speed 4.5 mph)
1 minute	Up interval—HR = 95% (Incline 6%—approx. speed 5.5+ mph)
2 minutes	Down interval—HR = 80% (Incline 1%—approx. speed 4.5+ mph)
Next 50 minutes	Repeat
5 minutes	Cooldown—HR = 65% (Incline 0%—approx speed 4.5+ mph)

Or

PETE'S AM TREADMILL WORKOUT

Warm-up	
5 minutes	HR = 70% to 80% (Incline 1—approx. speed 5.0)
Workout	
25 minutes	HR = 80% to 85% (Incline 2—approx. speed 5.5)
25 minutes	HR = 85% to 95% (Incline 2—approx. speed 6.5)
Cooldown	
5 minutes	HR = 70% to 80% (Incline 1—approx. speed 5.0)

and

PETE'S MIDNIGHT 20 TREADMILL WORKOUT

Warm-up	
2 minutes	HR = 70% to 85% (Incline 1—approx. speed 5.0)
Workout	
15 minutes	HR = 85% to 95% (Incline 2—approx. speed 7.5)
Cooldown	
3 minutes	HR = 70% to 85% (Incline 1—approx. speed 4.5)

WEEKS 9 TO 12
WEDNESDAY AND SATURDAY PRIMARY WORKOUT

PETE'S HIGHLY ADVANCED FINAL MONTH INTERVAL TREADMILL WORKOUT (TARGET HEART RATE AVERAGE 90% AND ABOVE)

HIGHLY ADVANCED!
1-hour incline sprints 2x per week
Incline 12 / Speed 10
2 minutes sprinting / 1 minute rest
Repeat for 1 hour

WEEKS 9 TO 12

WEDNESDAY AND SATURDAY SECONDARY WORKOUT

PETE'S A.M. TREADMILL WORKOUT

Warm-up	
5 minutes	HR = 70% (Incline 1—approx. speed 5.0)
Workout	
25 minutes	HR = 80% to 85% (Incline 2—approx. speed 5.5)
25 minutes	HR = 85% to 95% (Incline 2—approx. speed 6.5)
Cooldown	
5 minutes	HR = 70% to 80% (Incline 1—approx. speed 5.0)

FOREVER FUNDAMENTALS— STEP THREE CHECKLIST

NOW THAT YOU'VE STARTED LOSING THOSE POUNDS *FAST* IN STEP 3: Your Pursuit, you will be moving on to the maintenance stage— Step 4: Your Purpose. Answer the following questions about your Forever Habits to prepare you for what is to come.

MASTER YOUR MIND

Now that we will be relaxing your routine a little bit, which of the following Forever Habits will keep you focused on a healthy lifestyle?

- Daily journaling your journey in your LIF2 Success Journal
- Touching a teammate regularly

- Revising your team to reflect a new stage in life
- Repeating your Personal Success Statement
- Repeating your Personal Power Goals, the "top 3" of your Top 10
- Wearing your goal outfit on a regular basis
- Putting up photos of the "new" and "old" me together

MANAGE YOUR MOUTH

Now that your meal plans will be a little bit more flexible, as it was in Step 2: Your Plan, which of the following will help keep your Purpose meal plans healthy and honest?

- Eating within your goal weight Personal Daily Fuel Goal
- Looking up new foods in your handy carry-along calorie counter
- Revising your weekly food plan to allow more variety
- Creating a new grocery list and shopping list, while still living by the motto "If it's not on the list, I must resist."
- Bringing your own food to parties and celebrations
- Researching restaurant menus before going out to eat
- Teaching or terminating saboteurs
- Moving to water from diet sodas and juices

MULTIPLY YOUR MUSCLES

Now that your exercise time and intensity are going to come back to a *forever* level, which of the following will ensure you spend enough time working out to maintain that slim figure?

- Continuing to build muscle through regular resistance training
- Continuing to burn fat using ABC Circuits four times a week
- Continuing cardio exercise twice a week on Wednesday and Saturday
- Keeping track of workouts in your exercise log
- Developing a running or cycling program that keeps you working in your aerobic range
- Engaging in enjoyable activities on your "rest day" that keep you burning calories

Congratulations! You made it through the intense Pursuit step and you're moving on to Step 4: Your Purpose. Use your restored health and your newly developed Forever Habits to discover—or rediscover—your purpose in life. This is a time of celebration, without letting down our vigilance or becoming overconfident. Above all, this is a time to reach back and help someone else struggling with his or her weight. As you teach others, you will be reinforcing your own Forever Habits. Now let's move on!

STEP FOUR

YOUR PURPOSE

"LIF2 provides every detail needed to allow students to create an eating and exercise plan they can follow for the rest of their lives. There are no shortcuts, there are no gimmicks, just thorough, well-researched insights to help every student reach his or her weight loss goal. If you are looking for lasting results and a lifelong plan, LIF2 is for you."

—GEORGE, LIF2 STUDENT

"I have tried so many diet plans—more than I can count. What's different about LIF2 is that it is something you can do for the rest of your life. It's not a fad diet that's here today, gone tomorrow. It's a plan that can fit into your life. It's a plan that can change your life."

—KENDALL, LIF2 STUDENT

"LIF2 has helped me change my life. I'm not the same person I was when this year started. I may not be at my goal yet, but I know that I will get there. It's not just a dream anymore, I know that it's going to happen. Thank you for helping me to find my strength."

—AMY, LIF2 STUDENT

CHAPTER

18

MOVE INTO MAINTENANCE

WHAT WOULD BE THE FIRST THING YOU WOULD DO ON THE DAY AFTER you won the $100,000 At-Home Prize on *The Biggest Loser*? I mean the very first thing.

I went for an hour and a half run.

That's right, the very next morning after celebrating my $100,000 victory I woke up at 6:00 a.m. and went out for a ninety-minute run all by myself.

I can just hear what many of you might be saying: "Are you crazy?" Once I returned to the hotel, one of my fellow contestants, who had worked just as hard as I had to get ready for the finale, asked me, "Pete, don't you ever stop?"

To be honest, I did not answer her. I thought the question was really odd. To me this was not the end of the journey but rather the beginning. I had lost a ton of weight, and now it was time to start the next step of life: maintenance. Maintenance was not going to be as hard as losing, but it was not going to be easy either. It would require that I set new goals, adopt different habits, learn new skills, adjust my eating, find new mentors, endure new challenges, and test out what I had done in the maze called real life.

The answer to her question, of course, is "no." I am not going to stop. Ever. I'm not going to stop learning about this new healthy lifestyle. I'm not going to stop learning how to eat healthy foods. I'm not giving up on regular, rigorous exercise. No matter how hard things get, I am not going to stop. I am too valuable as a human being. I have too much to offer to my family and friends. I have too much to offer to the world. With everything that is within me, I will not stop and go back to that huge guy on the cover with all of his health issues and limitations. No matter how many times I slip, I won't stop. I can't stop.

And neither should you.

ENJOYING YOUR NEW LIFE

Congratulations! You made it through Step 3: Your Pursuit and you have started Losing It Fast. Combined with Step 1: Your Power and Step 2: Your Plan, you are on your way to truly losing it forever.

Now you've moved on to Step 4: Your Purpose, and you should be proud of yourself. I call this step Your Purpose because now that you're overcoming one of the major obstacles to happiness in this life—poor health—you are free to discover and focus in on your real purpose in life. It's time to use the success you've experienced in weight loss to drive your ambition in other areas. I have found that the same principles that allowed me to be successful in weight loss have translated into other areas of my life—being committed to changing what I say to myself about myself and my future, making powerful emotional goals, developing and relying on a team, having a daily plan that develops my consistent habits, modifying my behaviors to stay on plan, and having times when I aggressively practice those habits for faster results. These all apply to achieving my purpose in the bigger picture of life.

This is the step of life I am in currently, so I want you to know you have a teammate in the journey. I hope you feel like I did when I lost all my weight after *The Biggest Loser*. I thought to myself, "I'm never going back to that old life!"

When I was really heavy, I could gain five pounds and not even feel it. After I got thin, five extra pounds made me very uncomfortable. That's where you will be very soon. I want you to enjoy your new leaner self so much that you actually forget what it was like to be overweight. You don't have to go back to being heavy—that's what this step is all about.

So many programs help you lose weight and then leave you high and dry without teaching you to move into maintenance. That's why I designed a plan that is good for life, not just for a short-term weight loss. But to maintain your new, lean figure means you've got to stay on top of some things.

LEARNING TO FORGIVE YOURSELF

There is a wonderful song by Donnie McClurkin that goes, "We fall down, but we get up . . ." There is no better way to express what our attitude should be when we experience setbacks on the road to maintaining our health.

I said this before: Through this whole learning process, we need to learn to forgive ourselves and move past temporary failures. Avoid what I call the "cycle of death." That's when we have a bad lunch and we feel so bad about messing up that we end up having a bad dinner. That bad dinner means that we've blown it again, so why not have a late-night ice cream? Now that bad lunch has turned into a bad day all together. And that bad day can easily turn into a bad weekend, which ends up turning into a bad week.

The truth is, one bad lunch does not have to equal a bad dinner, a bad dinner does not have to equal a bad day, and a bad day does not have to equal a bad weekend. As I said before, if you had a flat tire, would you go around and puncture all the other tires on your car? Of course not. You spent too many calories on lunch—okay, forgive yourself for messing up immediately and adjust your next meal to make up for it and go on to lose that Forever Few you're shooting for.

Remember, we are not on a diet. We are living a new life. There's no quitting or giving up. When we encounter setbacks, we stand back up, dust ourselves off, and keep moving toward health and toward our life's purpose.

THE FIVE RS OF MAINTENANCE

Once you get to this point, you have two roads you can take. The first is the one many people take—you can become overconfident, regress, and go backward. Or you can take the gains that you have experienced and you can keep moving forward. Obviously, you need to keep moving forward. There is no such thing as standing still in this life.

I'm no stranger to stepping on the scale and seeing it move in the wrong direction, even after all this time. So whenever I start to struggle with my weight, in my own Purpose step, I practice what I call the Five Rs:

- Review
- Revise
- Repeat
- Reward
- Reach Back

If you practice these steps, instead of getting frustrated when things go wrong, you will quickly get back on track and avoid the cycle of death.

WHAT IS YOUR KRYPTONITE?

One of the primary problems with the maintenance stage is overconfidence. I call it the Superman complex. You start thinking, "Okay, I've got this thing down, I know what I'm doing. I don't need to really pay attention to this or that. I've got this! I can do anything!" And you're right, you can do anything, almost. If you have lost a substantial amount of weight, then that sense of accomplishment is well founded. But watch out, Superman or Superwoman—you, too, can be at the mercy of Kryptonite. In my case my Kryptonite was—you guessed it—food. And it is everywhere. What does a food addict do when the source of his addiction is all around him? Unlike many other addictions, I actually need a certain amount of food to survive. What I have to do is to constantly review how I am doing.

REVIEW

The first place you may be tempted to loosen up a little may be with your weekly weigh-in. It may take a while but, like me, you may say to yourself, "I've got this. I'll just weigh in once a month." Bad idea. If by chance you have not been on top of things over the last thirty days, then you will really be behind the eight ball if you wait for an entire month to weigh in. Just think about what can happen in thirty days—holiday parties, stress eating due to family and work situations, this and that and the other. Within thirty days you can actually lose so much ground that you may have to start all over and develop new habits. So I encourage you to continue weighing in once a week at a minimum, even during Your Purpose step. Then if you find things are going the wrong way, you go back and ask yourself, "What should I be doing to correct this?" My weigh-in day is every Tuesday morning. I suggest that if you haven't already, you pick a day of the week to weigh-in and stick to it.

A couple of years ago, a contestant from *The Biggest Loser* contacted me. She had been off the show for three or four years and she said, "So, what do you do for exercise?" I was in shock. I thought, "You have got to be kidding me. We had the best trainers on the planet tell us what to do. Now you're trying to figure out what to do for exercise? You should just be going back to the basics."

You need to do the same. Go back and review the basics. Most of these were taught in Step 1: Your Power and Step 2: Your Plan. Review the principles you've learned in these steps concerning your mind, your mouth, and your muscles. You've got everything you need right here to get and keep yourself headed in the right direction. All you have to do is review it and apply it.

It's also helpful to read magazine articles and blogs written by smart people on health and wellness. Reading is so important that it could be its own "R." When you do sit down and read, don't take just anyone's word, because there are some people who don't know your specific situation and goals. But we can always grow in our knowledge and add to our education. I subscribe to three monthly health magazines and a monthly nutrition newsletter; I also read health-related books as well as tons of blogs. If you're not a former food addict like me, you may not need to read quite this much, but remember, you need to take care of your health for the rest of your life. The battle is not over until you are, so keep learning. Knowledge is power—so use it to Lose It Forever!

REVISE

As I have stated, whenever I notice that I have gotten away from the basics I inevitably find the scale pushing in the wrong direction. I have learned from experience not to panic. I take an honest look at myself and revise some of my daily habits. I have learned, and this is important, that a bad day doesn't need to turn into a bad weekend, and a bad weekend doesn't need to turn into a bad week. If I catch it early and just revise some things, I pull myself back on track.

Sometimes you need to revise things by making some small changes in the way you're living. Are there foods that have crept back into your cupboard that you need to clear out? Have you started going for the refined carbs just before bedtime again? Maybe you need to revise your food or exercise habits as well as your schedule to get back to where you know you should be.

At times I have allowed certain foods to sneak back into my diet that I simply should not be eating. This has become one of my pet peeves with other short-term, fad, drastic diet programs—once you lose the weight, they let you go back to eating the same way that got you heavy in the first place!

It's easy to do. I would start saying to myself, "I have gotten more disciplined; I can have a little more cake around the house. I can buy these cookies for guests." Really? Are you sure about that? Think again.

I have this love affair with mayonnaise. Not light mayonnaise. I mean real, 100 percent full-calorie Hellmann's mayonnaise. I can put it on anything. In the old days, I used to dip potato chips in it. That's everything you need to gain weight: fat, salt, and fried food. I'm telling you, mayonnaise was a trigger food for me. It still is, I've discovered.

I know that because, over time, I have tried to talk to myself and say,

"I'm a stud. I can have mayonnaise in the house. Oh, look, five dollars for a big jar, that will last a month." Then the next week I would be up 2 pounds. What happened? That whole jar was missing. That was 7000 calories.

How did I consume 7000 calories over the course of a week? Mayonnaise was a trigger food, and I did not pay attention to what I was doing with it. Remember, a trigger food is any food that causes you to lose control and overeat in an unplanned and unhealthy way. I would put a little bit of mayo on anything I brought home. I would have a salad and be careful to put low-calorie dressing on it . . . as well as a couple of spoons of mayo. Baked chicken . . . and a little mayo. Everything had a little bit of mayo on it. So I had to take a look at myself and revise what I was eating again to get back to basics—and keep full-calorie mayo out of the house.

I have had to assess my exercise habits as well. Have you stopped creating a caloric deficit by exercising? Revise your routine and pick it back up. Have you become bored with working out at home by yourself? Revise your habits by joining a gym or taking classes with other people. Go back over your basics, revise what you are doing. That is a really key aspect of Your Purpose step—doing the right thing over and over and over.

You may also need to revise your exercise routine to reflect the new realities in your life. Use my Lose It Forever Weekly Maintenance Workout Plan, or come up with a plan of your own. The nice thing about this plan is that you will be doing enough resistance—twice a week—to keep the muscles strong, but you will be focused on the cardio side. This will allow you to get outdoors if you choose.

PETE THOMAS'S LOSE IT FOREVER WEEKLY MAINTENANCE WORKOUT PLAN

Note: When doing ABC Circuits, perform each exercise for one minute, then move to the next exercise in order. After you complete all three exercises in order (one circuit), then start over until you complete the circuit three times. Then move to the next circuit with as little rest as possible in between circuits.

Monday	60 + minutes of cardiovascular exercise at 80% of HR or higher (H.I.I.T. or LSD)					

	Circuit 1	**Circuit 2**	**Circuit 3**	**Circuit 4**	**Circuit 5**	**Cardio Circuit**
Tuesday	**A** Push-ups **B** Air Squats **C** Jumping Jacks	**A** Chest Presses with DB **B** Sumo Squats **C** Butt Kicks	**A** Anterior Raises with DB **B** Squat Hops **C** Up Downs (10 ct)	**A** Biceps Curls **C** Jumping Jacks **B** Sit-ups	**A** Hammer Curls **C** Butt Kicks **B** Plank	Up Downs (10 ct) Jumping Jacks Butt Kicks

Wednesday	60 + minutes of cardiovascular exercise at 80% of HR or higher (H.I.I.T. or LSD)					

	Circuit 1	**Circuit 2**	**Circuit 3**	**Circuit 4**	**Circuit 5**	**Cardio Circuit**
Thursday	**A** Dumbbell Row—left arm **B** Reverse Lunges **C** Mountain Climbers	**A** Dumbbell Row—right arm **B** Side Lunges **C** High Knees	**A** Supermans **B** Forward Static Lunge **C** Burpees	**A** Overhead Triceps Presses—left arm **C** Mountain Climbers **B** Bicycle Abs	**A** Overhead Triceps Presses—right arm **C** High Knees **B** Russian Twist Sit-ups	Burpees Mountain Climbers High Knees

Friday	60 + minutes of cardiovascular exercise at 80% of HR or higher (H.I.I.T. or LSD)					
Saturday	60 + minutes of cardiovascular exercise at 80% of HR or higher (H.I.I.T. or LSD)					
Sunday	Active Rest Day					

REPEAT

Hopefully, this will not shock you, but you will need to do the right things for about five to seven years before it becomes second nature. I'm serious about this. I believe that you should repeat the basics for a number of years before you start playing around and trying to add trigger foods back into your life. Here's why.

Challenges of Life

We have to go through life's challenges and seasons and react to them in a new way and repeat that success so it can become part of our "new normal."

The last few years have not been a breeze for me. Winning $100,000 does not make your problems go away. I have had several serious challenges, like everyone else. However, I have learned over time not to turn to food for comfort. Instead I will go to the gym and put in an exhausting workout or, best of all, cry out to God in prayer. You have to find some way to get the frustration out without burying your sorrows in a gallon of chocolate-chocolate-chip ice cream. Take a dance class or some other recreational class. Take up kickboxing. Personally, I'm afraid I would break the equipment, but that might be a way for you to work out your tension. I had a student who took a fifty-mile bike ride when he needed to clear his head. The point is, this habit of turning to food can be replaced over time when healthy actions are repeated.

I am not saying that you can't have snacks. Hopefully you have already modified the kind of snacks that you're eating. I'm talking about staying away from the old, sugary, calorie-filled snacks that you used to keep around your house when you know that they are trigger foods. Let's leave them out of the house for a few years until you develop a certain amount of discipline. Believe me, you will really only be able to handle it after a few years of doing without it.

What we're trying to do here is actually replace your memories, and that takes time. I can hardly remember the old days, when I needed a lap belt extender on an airplane. I have forgotten what it feels like to have to sit at a table in a restaurant because I couldn't fit in a booth. I have literally replaced my memories by repeating new behaviors over and over and over. Weight gain makes me uncomfortable now, so I'm willing to give up those things that are bad for me. That kind of thought process takes repetition. Sometimes it takes a lot of repetition practiced over a long time.

The other thing that repetition will do is train us to find our comfort in the right place. Those of us who belong to the More Food or More Flavor Families often look to food for comfort, which is one reason we were so heavy in the first place. Now you have to consciously start looking to other things for comfort. I want you to get to the point where you feel so good about yourself, you are so confident with yourself, that you don't turn to food for comfort.

After you repeat the basics over and over again, I want you to plan something special for yourself because you are doing some amazing things.

REWARD

Part of successful, healthy living is learning to put *your* needs first. That may sound selfish to you, but part of the reason you became heavy in the first place may be because you put everyone else's needs above your own. Now that you've lost the weight, you really need to look at what you are doing as a blessing and a benefit to your family, to your friends, to your work colleagues, everybody around you. So, as you invest in yourself with a new healthy lifestyle, reward yourself. There is nothing wrong with treating yourself with that fancy new dress, new sports equipment, a weekend away, or whatever. You hit a weight loss goal, you deserve to reward yourself.

REACH BACK

Now that you have come to this point of health and success in your life, it is time to help someone else. In my experience of being around and talking to very successful people, most of them can barely explain the basic principles that they used to become successful, let alone teach them to others. It is not a character flaw. It is just that the things they practice daily are second nature, so they've forgotten that they ever had to work for them.

I have asked you to maintain a LIF2 Success Journal, for several reasons. One is that people who journal have been found to be exponentially more successful than those who don't. Another is so that you won't forget what caused *you* to be successful. You can go back and read your journal to see how far you've come, and what steps you took to get to where you are today.

One of the primary principles shared by those who are most successful in all areas of life is the principle of *paying it forward*. Some call it sowing or just simply giving. Others call it teaching one another. I call it reaching back.

Throughout this program I have encouraged you to celebrate each and every success by going to www.PeteThomas.com and trumpeting your success. I call this touching a teammate. This is not about bragging or boasting, even though I do want you to be proud of your accomplishments. Rather, it is about giving back to others. The purpose of celebrating in public is to reach out or encourage someone else who may be struggling along the path to health.

Many of us have suffered through the trials of weight loss and regain. Can you pay it forward by taking a couple of minutes of your time to talk about your success? Even if it is as simple as saying, "Another Forever Five gone" or "Another Forever Habit established," this alone will revive someone who may have lost all hope that they can lose weight forever. If you want to share more detail about how a certain principle changed the way you think or act, that would be an even greater help to others. Studies have shown that you retain only a fraction of what you hear or see or read if you don't act on it, but when you teach something to others, you retain over 90 percent of the information. In other words, helping others will actually help you. In short, I want you to reach out to others by sharing your success. I strongly suggest that you buy this book for someone else close to you, or at least recommend it on your social media sites. That would be another "R"—recommend—but I'm going to quit while I'm ahead.

So those are the Five Rs of the Purpose step:

- **Review** what you are doing and review the principles that made you successful in the first place; writing in your journal will help this process.
- **Revise** and correct those things that have caused you to slip back.
- **Repeat** those things that are successful and build new memories.
- **Reward** yourself for a job well done.
- **Reach back** to others by sharing your successful experiences.

YEARLY RITUAL

I wear the same suit to every one of my final classes when I teach my in-person weight loss course. It's the suit I wore when I won the At-Home Prize on *The Biggest Loser* finale in Season 2. It still fits.

I don't wear it to relive my fifteen minutes of fame. I wear it because it's both a goal and a reward for me. It's a goal because I need to keep myself slim enough to wear it in front of my students; it's a reward because it gives me an amazing feeling of accomplishment to be able to put it on year after year. The only way that I am able to wear it seven years later is because I practice the things I have taught you in this book.

I want you to consider setting a yearly goal. At a certain point every year—maybe on New Year's Eve—you are going to fit into that dynamite outfit no matter what. Maybe it's a certain bathing suit for summer vacation, or an Easter outfit in the spring. I hope you realize by now that it is very important for you to set these kinds of goals.

STAY CONNECTED

Let me repeat something I've said several times in this book: Weight loss is not something you can do alone! So stay connected with us, even as you live in the Purpose step of your weight loss journey. Please come to the website and tell us your story, or as I like to say, "touch a teammate." Your story is going to help encourage someone else. Read the stories of others, so that you can continue to walk in the health you've achieved.

I'm proud of you. You did what no one—including you, probably—thought you could do. Now go and help someone else take back his or her life, one Forever Habit at a time.

A STORY STILL BEING WRITTEN

Do you know who you are? Have you discovered your real purpose in life? I have shared many of my early struggles in these pages. I did this not to draw attention to myself but because they have shaped who I am and my subsequent struggles with food and obesity. I believe one of the reasons I experienced certain challenges in life is so that I would be able to show others that God can use our struggles to point us toward our life's ultimate purpose. Allow me to share another such story with you.

In my early twenties I joined a church called Labor of Love Ministries in Ann Arbor, Michigan. This was a very unsettling time for me, as I had dropped out of college and was trying to find my way in life. The insecurities of my youth would come through regularly in the gruff and abrupt way I would interact with people. I was insecure about my past and scared of the future. I remember being in church during one service and raising my hands to thank God for this or that and I actually banged my hands on the ceiling of this little church. I was so embarrassed that I refused to raise my hands above my shoulders for months. Then one day the shortest minister in the church came over to pray for me and he said, "Stand up! God made you tall!" I had never heard or even considered that before. I wondered to myself, "If God made me tall, then maybe he made me other things as well. And maybe he wants me to do something in particular with my life." I was soon on a quest to learn what God wanted me to do in my life.

Not long after starting this quest I was sitting in church and received an amazingly powerful mental impression telling me that I was to become a speaker, teacher, and athlete. This impression was so strong that I knew it was from God, but I did not know how to act on it. Our church was full of so many highly educated people that I was intimidated to speak up in open Bible study discussions. I was not enrolled in school, so I was unlikely to become a certified teacher, and I had never played sports in school, so I could not see myself becoming a professional athlete. While I knew that this was a message directly to me from God, all I could do was simply file it away in my memory bank for future consideration.

Over the next few years I set about improving my education by attending classes at the local community college and reading the Bible, as well as material on other religions. My knowledge of and faith in a real God deepened and I felt my insecurities fall off. Over the years I even went on to become successful in different business endeavors while keeping the idea of becoming a speaker, teacher, and athlete filed away in the back of my mind.

Amazingly enough, here we are today, over twenty years after when I first heard God tell me I was going to be a speaker. I now regularly travel across the country to speak to company executives and their employees as I help launch corporate wellness programs. Through this book and my seminars, classes, and boot camps, I am able to be a teacher to those who are weeding through the mountains of health and wellness information and misinformation. And on a regular basis I participate in athletic events such as a two-hundred-mile relay race, a one-hundred-mile bicycle race, triathlons, a full marathon, and a half marathon every single year on my birthday.

I am here because one day in my early twenties I heard the message of a perfect and loving God who desired a relationship with me. I have come to understand that even in the midst of my health struggles God had a plan to set me on the path toward his purpose for my life. As I sit here typing, my desire is that these words will instill a sense of hope in you. Weight loss and good health are not an end unto themselves. Rather they are simply a step toward fulfilling your ultimate destiny and purpose in life. Think of it this way: Your physical body is simply the cup that carries your life's purpose. Just like a cracked or broken-down cup cannot properly fulfill its function and hold its contents, if your body is broken down, then you cannot complete your life's purpose.

So I dedicate this book to you, the reader, and to your good health—and ultimately your purpose in life. I thank God for *The Biggest Loser,* not simply because it ultimately saved my life, but because through it I can help save someone else's life. Take my experiences and my knowledge, and use them to regain your health or discover good health for the first time. Then let's begin writing the story of the rest of your unique life.

KEY POINTS

- Through this whole learning process, we need to learn to forgive ourselves and move past temporary failures.
- Whenever you start to struggle with your weight, practice the Five Rs:
  - Review
  - Revise
  - Repeat
  - Reward
  - Reach back
- What we're trying to do is actually replace your memories, and that takes time.
- Weight loss is not something you can do alone! So stay connected with your team, even as you live in the Purpose step of your weight loss journey.

CHAPTER 18 CHALLENGES

New Challenges | Remember the Five Rs

We need to remember to review, revise, repeat, reward, and reach back to others for the rest of our lives. If we do that, we'll continue to walk in the new health we've achieved.

Mentor Someone

You'll really cement these principles when you teach them to someone. You'll also pay closer attention to your own habits, as you've set yourself up as a model.

Keep Celebrating!

You've done an amazing job. Keep periodically rewarding yourself (with healthy rewards) for a job well done!

Ongoing Challenges | Weigh Yourself Weekly

Don't get overconfident and weigh yourself less often. It takes work to maintain your new lean body.

Stay Connected

Touch a teammate at www.PeteThomas.com. Your triumph may help others overcome hurdles in their own journey.

INDEX

Goals, 10. (*cont.*)
  saboteurs of, 55
  S.M.A.R.T., 24–28, 30–31
  specific, 25
  statements and, 28–29
  supporters of, 55
  teammates helping, 53
  time-based, 27–28
  for weight loss, 24–28, 146–47
  workouts influenced by, 146–47
God
  food made by, 87
  story involving, 304–6
Groceries
  list, 127–29, 130–31
  for meal plan, 127–31
  nutrition labels of, 129–30
  scavenger hunt, 132–33
Gyms, 163–64

Habits
  checklist, 58, 218–19, 287–88
  eating, 110–11
  exercise, 152, 299
  food influencing, 17–18
  goals influenced by, 30–31
  revision of, 298–99
  success, 89, 102, 142
  systematic education forming, 7–8
  weight loss influenced by, 219
Hamstring, 267–71
Harper, Bob, 200
Heart rate, 147–48
  on *The Biggest Loser*, 179
  formulas, 205
  Michaels influencing, 201
  monitor, 210, 211
  running, during, 210, 211–12
  training, 204–5
  weight loss influenced by, 179
HFCS. *See* High fructose corn syrup
High-fructose corn syrup (HFCS), 86–87
High-intensity circuit resistance training, 179–81, 187–97
  circuits, 234
  exercises, 251–80
High-intensity interval training (H.I.I.T.), 157–58, 172
  examples, 168–71
  workouts, 169–71, 173, 233
H.I.I.T. *See* High-intensity interval training
Holappa, Matt, 200–201
Hormones
  bad, 108–9

carbohydrates blocking, 115
  description of, 95, 106
  good, 107–8
  insulin as, 94–96
  sugar releasing, 91
  undereating influencing, 82

In-N-Out Burger, 135
Injury, resistance training preventing, 176
Insulin
  as hormone, 94–96
  response, 94–96, 231–32
  weight loss influenced by, 109
Intensity
  on *The Biggest Loser*, 150
  of workouts, 147–48

"Jacquata" (LIF2 student), 23
"Jennifer" (LIF2 student), 198
"Jessica" (LIF2 student), 61
"Jim" (LIF2 student), 90
Journal
  calories in, 77
  on carbohydrates, 98–99, 103
  on commitment, 20
  on exercise, 153, 178, 183–84
  food, 9, 17–18, 21
  goals in, 30–31
  meal plan in, 122
  reason for, 302
  Road Map to Success in, 173
  S.M.A.R.T. goals in, 30–31
  statement in, 31
  on workouts, 197
Joyce, Monica, 200–201

Kaizen (little changes making difference), 86
"Katie" (LIF2 student), 174
"Keith" (LIF2 student), 236
"Kendall" (LIF2 student), 11, 293
Knowledge
  of muscle groups, 188
  reading to increase, 297–98
  of weight loss, 19–20, 125–26
  of workouts, 188

Lactate threshold, 208–9
Levine, Jeffrey, 46–47, 160, 182, 230
LIF2 Success Journal. *See* Journal
Life, 294–95, 300–302
"Lisa" (LIF2 student), 223
Lists. *See also* Checklists
  equipment, 21–22

Obesity
  death caused by, 15
  sugar causing, 97
Overconfidence, 296–97
Overeating, 64
  Daily Fuel Goal, 65–66
  weight influenced by, 65–66

Pain, 162–63
  knee, 206–7
  muscle, 182–83
  running, 205–7
Parties, 138–39, 142
The Passion of the Christ, 79–80
Paying it forward, 302–3
Perfect Personalized Forever Meal Plan. *See* Meal
    plan
Perfect Personalized Forever Workout Plan.
    See Workout plans
Perfect Personalized Fuel Plan. *See* Fuel plan
Peripheral heart action (PHA), 180–81
Personal Daily Fuel Goal. *See* Daily Fuel Goal
Personal Power Goals. *See* Goals
Personal Success Statements. *See* Statements
PHA. *See* Peripheral heart action
Pictures
  before, 29, 31
  of goal outfit, 31
Pigg, Mike, 204
Protein
  calories burned by, 102
  importance of, 99
Public
  as team, 38–39

Quadriceps, 271–74

Reaching back, 302–3
Reading, 297–98
Rebound effect, undereating causing, 76
Repetition, 300–302
Rest, body allowed to recover by, 110
Rest days, 193–94
Resting metabolic rate (RMR). *See* Daily Fuel
    Goal
Reviewing, 297–98
Revision, 296–300
  of habits, 298–99
Rewards, 228–29, 307
  food as, 61–62, 139–40
  for goals, 29–30, 302
  system, 33
RMR. *See* Resting metabolic rate
Road Map to Success

creating, 173
journaling, 173
"Rodney" (LIF2 student), 185
Run-Walk-Run method, 204
Runners, 207–9
Running, 198
  benefits of, 199
  body adjusting to, 206–7
  classes, 200–201, 203, 215
  description of, 199
  heart rate during, 210, 211–12
  medical permission for, 206, 215
  methods, 204–5
  mind influencing, 202
  as motivation, 214–15
  pain, 205–7
  plans, 209–12
  shoes, 200, 210, 211
  styles, 207–9
  time, 203, 215
  walking and, 205
  weight loss influenced by, 208–9

Salt, 91–92
  Michaels on, 100
  weight loss killed by, 100, 231
Set plans, 71, 72, 231
"Seth" (teammate), 47
Shoes, 200, 210, 211
Shoulders, 258
Shrimp, 101
S.M.A.R.T. goals, 24–28
  in journal, 30–31
Snacks
  discipline influencing, 301
  in meal plan, 119
  as trigger foods, 301
  weight loss influenced by, 110–11
Social networks, weight influenced by, 42
Sorrells, Shay, 15
Soul Food, 23
Squats, 271–74
Statements
  goals and, 28–29
  in journal, 31
  mind influenced by, 28–29
  reviewing, 78, 184
Steady state exercise, 155–57, 172
  workouts, 171, 173, 233
"Stephanie" (LIF2 student), 3
"Steve" (LIF2 student), 79
Strength of teammates, 50
Stress, time for relieving, 19, 21
Stretches, 165–68, 216, 238

Success
  Forever Few, 89
  habits, 89, 102, 142
  Road Map to, 173
  sharing, 303
  weight loss, 142, 216, 302–3
Sugar
  body poisoned by, 95–96
  fuel released by, 96
  high, 91
  hormones released by, 91
  obesity caused by, 97
  weight loss influenced by, 100, 231
  workouts influenced by, 93
Sugar substitutes. *See* Artificial sweeteners
Superman complex, 296–97
S.W.A.T. teammates, 46
Swimming
  time, 214
  for weight loss, 213–14
Systematic education, 7–8, 62

Teaching teammates, 50–52
Teammates, 42
  accountability, 43–44
  availability of, 50
  on *The Biggest Loser*, 46–47, 230
  choosing, 49–50
  contract signed by, 52–53
  encouragement, 43, 46–47
  food, 45
  goals helped by, 53
  online, 48–49, 230–31
  roles assigned to, 55–56
  spiritual, 47–48
  strengths of, 50
  S.W.A.T., 46
  teaching, 50–52
  as team, 39–40
  temperament of, 49
  terminating, 230
  touching, 302–3, 304
  trainers as, 44–45, 229–30
  weaknesses of, 50
  work, 48
  workout, 44–45
Teams
  accountability provided by, 38–40
  on *The Biggest Loser*, 34–38, 41–42, 230
  building, 42, 55
  communication with, 53, 78, 184
  connection to, 304, 307
  discipline and, 38, 40
  encouragement provided by, 41–42

large group as, 39
list and, 53, 55–56
mentor as, 39–40
public as, 38–39
rearranging, 53–54
social influence of, 42
teammate as, 39–40
terminations from, 230
trainer as, 39–40
weight loss influenced by, 37–38
yourself as, 40
Temptation foods, 34–36
Time
  on *The Biggest Loser*, 150
  calendar, put into, 21
  commitment to, 16–17
  for exercise, 18–19
  goals based on, 27–28
  running, 203, 215
  for stress relief, 19, 21
  swimming, 214
  weight loss and, 14–17
  weight loss influenced by, 226–27
  for workouts, 148–52
Torres, Dara, 214
Trainers, 164
  as team, 39–40
  as teammates, 44–45, 229–30
Trans fats, 100
Triceps, 259–60
Trigger foods, 299, 301
Type, 152–53

Undereating, 75–76
  hormones influenced by, 82
Upper back, 260–62
USDA. *See* Department of Agriculture, U.S.

Vegetables, caloric checkbook and, 125
Venuto, Tom, 38–40
VO$_2$ max, 209

Walking
  as exercise, 21
  running and, 205
Water, 164–65
  calories burned by, 232
Weakness
  of teammates, 50
Weight
  calories influencing, 65–66, 67
  exercise, used in, 176
  initial, 31–32
  killing, 104–5